evolution

OF COCOONS

evolution

OF COCOONS

A MOTHER'S

JOURNEY

THROUGH HER

DAUGHTER'S

BIPOLAR AND

ASPERGER'S

JANNA VOUGHT

Published by Familius LLC, www.familius.com

Familius books are available at special discounts for bulk purchases for sales promotions, family or corporate use. Special editions, including personalized covers, excerpts of existing books, or books with corporate logos, can be created in large quantities for special needs. For more information, contact Premium Sales at 559-876-2170 or email specialmarkets@familius.com

Library of Congress Catalog-in-Publication Data

2013942878

pISBN 978-1-938301-86-5
eISBN 978-1-938301-87-2

Printed in the United States of America

Edited by Victoria Candland
Cover Design by David Miles
Book design by Laurie Duersch

10 9 8 7 6 5 4 3 2 1

First Edition

Table of Contents

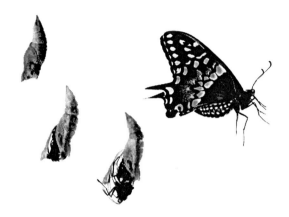

Introduction

Butterflies emerge from their cocoons perfect specimens of nature. Their wings display images of symmetry. The figures, colors, and designs on both wings are identical, each an exact replica of the other. Even the smallest spot, a fleck of color in the iris of the eye, appears on both sides, woven from the intricate layering of minute scales that fashion these masterpieces of art and marvels of creation. Such a natural ideal provides proof that living entities form as a result of ordered and predestined creation, not a series of random or unconscious coincidences.

Butterflies don't fly the same. Some, like the monarch, whose migration pattern requires flying great distances, have large broad wings that allow them to coast along in thermal uplifts with little exertion, while other species, like the viceroy, have small wings suited for rapid fluttering as their life cycle does not require them to travel far. Evolution dictates the formation of their wing and body design. Wings vary in shape, color, and function based upon the genetic makeup of the species as determined by their need to adapt to unique environments. Survival depends upon their wings, features vital for their prosperity.

Nature, however it strives for perfection, makes mistakes and creates small hiccups in the patterns. Anomalies in its design lead to devastation. Sometimes, monarchs emerge from their cocoon with crinkled or deformed wings. Several factors contribute to this debilitating condition: parasites, improperly formed chrysalis, disease. When this occurs, little hope remains for the creature; it cannot fly, and therefore, cannot survive. When encountering a deformed butterfly, one should consider destroying it in order to prevent the disease from spreading to the rest of the population. Placing the butterfly in a plastic bag in the freezer terminates its life; it's the humane thing to do.

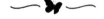

The Monarch's Fall

A Monarch fell
onto my bare foot
in the yard. Unfazed
by its plummet, wings crumpled
like tissue paper, it rolled to the side
in search of some greater
comfort. I nudged it
with my toe. The wings never
fluttered. It continued
on its way, stumbling over clumps
of brown grass, determined
to get somewhere, undaunted.
It lumbered over obstacles,
twisted wings dangling
behind: garden hose, tennis ball
relic used for canine leisure,
past rose bushes, unspoiled clover
blossom, the vegetable garden.
Exhausted by its trek
across the landscape,
it collapsed in filtered shadows
of the silver maple.

Others strum air with their wings.
They lift blue sky
where sunlight rides the wind.
Fast and sharp they glide, a million
patterns of perfect symmetry
take flight. Far from anywhere,
emptied of its last drops
of life, the butterfly brushed
its deformed wings against
my cupped hand. I plucked it
from the grass, studied
its silhouette in fading light.
With the last meticulous
fold of its wings, it shuddered
against an unseen chill and died,
destination never realized.
Is this what it feels like
when dreams die?
I buried its ply body
underneath a honeysuckle bush
ripe with new blooms and cried.

Her Arrival

November 18, 1998
4:31 p.m., a baby girl
6 pounds 8 ounces
20 inches

I had you
one afternoon, autumn days
dwindling into winter,
breeze brisk, sky smeared
with white cirrus. Kinetic energy
of bodies ignited formed
you. You bloomed. Eight months
and twenty-seven days
you drifted in liquid darkness
while I waited to greet you.

I didn't recognize
myself, feet far removed
from my body. My belly
stretched like a plastic bag
weighted with stones.
You moved away
from me like peeling fruit
from the rind.

You existed an endless
repetition of echoes,
a thousand lifetimes
exposed in your blue-
gray eyes. The life I owned
a tapestry of miscues
and imperfections until you.
My enormous body purged
of your being, belly soft
and empty. On a mild evening
in November, sky clinging
to light, I held you
to the sky so God
may greet you.

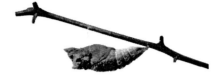

I.

"Life is nothing but a series of crosses for us mothers."

—*Collete*

My daughter is mentally ill. It sounds more like a confession than a proclamation, a dirty secret kept hidden from prying eyes, but I find no shame in admitting my reality. Destiny presented me with a situation that affords me access to a most strange, sometimes frightening, beautiful, and always intriguing world. Many never breech the barriers of this domain; they linger just outside the gates, afraid to enter. Others never find the opening, their presumptions obscuring their vision. I'm one of the lucky ones. God granted me access the day my daughter, Kamryn, entered the world.

Fate dealt Kamy a cruel hand, crippling her mind with a toxic brew of mental illnesses that destroy her capability to lead a regular life, that torture her spirit with anxiety, compulsions, hallucinations, and rage. As a result, our family endures the travails of her diseases. Instead of going to soccer games and dance recitals, we attend therapy sessions and medicine checks. We do not plan for college, but prepare for institutionalization.

We sign our daughter up for Social Security benefits while other parents register for swim classes or day camp. Local hospitals and the police are permanent fixtures on our speed dial. Our definition of normal lies just this side of deviancy. What others find abnormal is our reality.

The parents of a mentally ill child differ little from parents of healthy children. We weep, laugh, struggle, falter, endure—survive. What makes parenting unique for us, however, lies in the perpetual reminder of our undoing. Each day, we witness the devastation of our child as a result of his or her illness. Like the father who watches his child fade from cancer or the shock of a mother who loses her child to a violent crime, we spiral down, plummeting into misery only to rise again—a spirit resurrected. We live with the constant reminder of what we once had. Our therapist told us when we received Kamryn's diagnoses: "Grieve for your loss. The Kamryn you once knew is gone. You lost the life you knew before. All that you thought true is no more. You packed for Italy, but arrived in Holland."

We are a small family. Steve, Kamryn, our younger daughter Jordan, and I live in a modest brick house in the heart of Colorado Springs, a city nestled in the shadow of the Rocky Mountains. We function as a close-knit family. We experience each other's every triumph and failure, elation and despair. Steve and I always considered growing our family after Jordan's birth, something that I now am thankful never came to fruition. This family offers plenty. I maintain some semblance of a normal existence in our home, no doubt a daunting task. I had to overcome my need to control every aspect of life when Kamryn succumbed to her illnesses seven years ago.

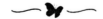

My first moments with Kamy did not provide me with any clues as to what lay before me. She looked and acted like any other healthy newborn: bright, attentive, wide-eyed in wonder to the world surrounding her tiny space. As she flourished into a beautiful little girl, she still seemed as average a child as any other. Sure, we had moments with her, but I attributed them to typical toddler issues that any first-time mother frets over: her lack of interest in playing with other children, food intolerance, separation anxiety, strange nightmares. My mother, friends, and pediatrician assured me to take heart; she would outgrow all of these behaviors with time, flourishing into a well-developed, high-functioning child. I believed them, for a while.

As time progressed, Kamy's behavior became more erratic, destructive, and concerning. She developed digestive issues associated with severe anxiety, performed the same ritualistic behaviors constantly, rejected any physical contact, even from me. She spoke of voices in her head, which she called her criminal friends that caused her to act inappropriately. Kamy refused to leave the house, flew into unprovoked rages at a moment's notice, purging herself of anger in the form of physical violence. At seven, she pleaded with my husband to keep a gun by our bed in case anyone broke into the house and tried to kill us. She could not eat a meal without vomiting due to her extreme anxiety. Things spiraled out of control, our family helpless to the invisible demons ravaging her body and mind. Our answer finally came when, at eleven, therapists and psychologists saddled my daughter with the most unimaginable burden. Finally, after so many years, our enemies revealed themselves, and for the first time in her life, I understood what my daughter, and my family, faced.

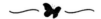

Kamy suffers from bipolar I disorder with psychotic tendencies, a brain disorder that affects her ability to regulate moods within a normal range. The severe symptoms debilitate. Kamy's manic cycling is dramatic and unstable, sometimes swinging across the emotional arc several times a week as opposed to the three or four episodes a year endured by those diagnosed with bipolar II. Kamy rides an emotional roller coaster every day, spiraling through dark tunnels, rocketing up steep inclines, plummeting into chasms, her illnesses relentless. The psychosis stems from hallucinations and delusions suffered during her manic and depressive phases. Her delusions are so real that it is impossible to reason with her. *No, Kamy, no one poisoned the water. No, Kamy, cutting up someone with the kitchen knife is not funny. Yes, Kamy, I am positive nothing is knocking at your window. Yes, Kamy, you may watch The Avengers for the thirteenth time in a week. No, Kamy, eating smoked meat will not kill you. Please, Kamy, tell your brain to quiet down, take a rest.*

Kamy's other major illness, Asperger's syndrome, is a developmental disorder that falls under the umbrella diagnosis of autism spectrum disorders. Asperger's is distinct from other forms of autism along the spectrum in many ways. People who suffer from Asperger's do not possess the limited cognitive development of those who suffer from autism, but they still grapple with stunted social and emotional development. Individuals with Asperger's suffer a myriad of crippling issues that prohibit their assimilation into mainstream society: obsessive thoughts and behaviors, repetitive rituals, inappropriate social behavior due to problems with non-verbal cues and expression, odd speech and language patterns, and a lack of coordinated motor skills. Because of the difficulties that result from their autism spectrum disorder, individuals with Asperger's syndrome fail to interact effectively with the outside world.

Kamy lives in a concrete world. Abstract concepts, including emotions, confuse her apathetic mind. She exhibits repetitive patterns of behavior and interests associated with

Asperger's. She adheres to strict routines so as not to disrupt the soothing stimuli such behavior provides; change terrifies her. Kamy stumbles about in her life, always one step behind the rest. Any activity requiring adeptness of motor skills provides a monumental challenge to her limbs that seem to move independently from the rest of her body. Each day presents a new difficulty for Kamy to overcome, be it emotional, physical, or mental; there is no reprieve.

Kamy also carries the diagnoses of general anxiety disorder and expressive-receptive language disorder, or Apraxia of speech. Her doctors and therapists often quip that she is a diagnostic text with arms and legs. Every day she fights against forces trapped inside her own mind. Imagine having no control over your thoughts and feelings—no release, no surrender. Kamryn walks these shadowed corridors, locked inside her ruination. No order exists in her world. She dwells in chaos; therefore, we do as well. We witness daily the loss of our daughter. As the curtain of mental illness closes over her gaze, so does it fall on any notion of our once perceived future. The day we learned her diagnoses forever changed our lives; it remains chiseled in my mind.

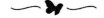

How We Got the News

This is the time
when your throat thickens,
hands turn to clay. Anxiety buzzes
around you like a late August fly fat
on sin and shit, refusing
to die. Ignore it;

it won't go away.
Inch your way down
the interstate, hope a horrific
accident causes a pileup,
derails your arrival.
You and your husband
sit in the parking lot
holding hands, refuse

each other's gaze.
Climb concrete steps
of this industrial building, gray
scar marring sky.
I have to go to the bathroom.
Make a charge past a sink
bank toward the solitary stall.
Crouch over the toilet, will
yourself to pee, take a moment
to calm ascending bile.
Your husband waits
outside, holds your purse
like a grenade

set for detonation.
Return to the hallway, lost
in an urban Amazon;
rubber Ficus and plastic plants
with stiff green spindles camouflage
walls. Feet find their way
along the known path:
hang a left at the dental office,
past a podiatrist and sport and spine
clinic, step inside the dark
interior and close

the door behind you.
She waits, arms folded,
for you, the parents, to arrive.
This is it: Try
not to cry.
"Are you ready?"
she asks. Nod your head
in affirmation. Now
you never can say no,
I'm not ready.

I hate this building. I hate the gray walls the color of week-old snow. I hate the linoleum stairs with their calico pattern that resembles regurgitated confetti. I hate the institution carpet–lined hallways. I hate the smell of pink wholesale bathroom soap infused with a tinge of dirty toilets and jasmine room freshener, a sickening concoction of beauty and waste. I hate the instrumental version of Elton John's "Tiny Dancer" wafting through the emptiness. I hate the closed steel doors that line the hallway like stern soldiers who stand guard to assure no prisoner escapes their confines. I hate this building; I hate this day.

Steve and I walk to the office three doors down the hallway on the right. We take the stairs instead of the drafty elevator; it takes more time to reach our destination. I occupy myself with innocuous thoughts as we wander down the shadowed corridor: *What should I make for dinner tonight? Are the roads going to be slick when we leave? How do I stop myself from crying?* We arrive at our destination. A small brass plate on the outside of the gray metal door bears the etching of a name: *Dr. Linda Thede, PsyD.* Steve looks at me and sighs; resolve weighs heavy in his blue eyes. "Let's go." I grab his arm; four tiny words infiltrate my daze: *Please, God, help us.* Steve thrusts his hand against the door, the barrier between this world and the next, between our today and whatever, and we step inside.

We enter the office and steer ourselves into a waiting room that adjoins the entrance. Navy upholstered chairs with rigid spines line the walls of the small space; a giant tawny colored bear sits perched on the floor, its head droops to one side in a display of defeat suffered at the hand of too many tight fisted blows to its cotton belly. I wonder if it's exhausted from listening to the family secrets and personal tribulations whispered into its tattered ears. I lay my coat in one of the empty chairs and sit down next to it. Steve, his hands buried in the front pockets of his jeans, wanders over to a wall filled with bro-chures: *Living with Autism, You and Your Schizophrenic Child, How to Recognize the Signs of Depression, What is Bipolar Disorder?* He selects a title that piques his interest and sits down next to me. We sit in silence—waiting.

I stare down at the carpet; the imprints of all those who sat here before me are buried into the worn pile. My sneakered toe traces the pattern of unknown footprints as I imagine what they look like. Were their eyes downcast like mine as they real-ized their shock, wonderment, and lack of understanding: *How did we get here? What happened? What do we do now?* I know these questions well, for they swirl about my head in a tireless evolu-tion. I feel kinship with the lost souls that haunt this space. The tired and the isolated, sequestered from the rest for one shift in a variable, one slip of the chromosome, one moment when God turned away.

The door from the inner office down the hall swings open and brings me back into the room, away from my inner space. A man and woman emerge into the hallway. The woman clutches a crumpled tissue in one hand, a purse in the other. The man walks two steps behind, his shoulders curved down in a defeated slump. They glance into the waiting room where we sit, observers to their pain. I want to run, to push past them in my escape, but I don't. I sit with my feet cemented in place, and stare. With the brief lock of our gazes, we are kindred souls, if only for that one hiccup in time. The man holds the outer door open for the woman and they shamble out into the dying light.

Seconds later, another figure appears in the doorway of the waiting room. My heart skips a beat at the sight of her: *Here we go.* A plump woman appears, dressed in khaki pants and a cream turtleneck. A topaz and gold paisley scarf weaves its way in a casual manner around her neck and her dark blond hair is swept up in a clip. She smiles at us and waves, "Steve and Janna, why don't you come on back? We have a lot to discuss today."

"Hello, Dr. Thede," we mumble in unison as we rise from our chairs and follow her down the hallway like petulant children summoned to the principal's office, heads hanging, feet shuffling. The walls along our path are tattooed with drawings, paintings, and colorings of various scenes: a stick figure family gathered under a rainbow, floating trees, lavender unicorns with bleeding eyes, black clouds spilling angry rain, a little girl standing alone—crying. I wonder what truths hide beneath the layers of wax and lead, what untold mysteries of the human psyche unfurl themselves in the intricate artwork of the mentally ill? Do I want to know? We reach the door to her office. She presses against the door and ushers us inside.

A large picture window exposes the expanse of the interstate that runs behind the building. The clouds hang low and heavy. A copper fountain on top of a glass credenza spills water over a meticulously arranged pile of river rock, its bubbles bursting over the granite with tinkles of liquid laughter. The ambient noise it creates drowns out the mumbled conversations between patient and self, mother and daughter, husband and wife. A large desk fashioned from polished wood sits in front of the window with file folders and various papers scattered on the surface. I wonder if I can see the dark rings under my eyes in my reflection in the surface.

Dr. Thede sits down in a leather wingback chair and motions for us to sit across from her. "Have a seat." I wedge myself into the cushions of a sofa that appears crafted from remnants of curtain fabric circa the 1800's. Its heavy velour dyed the shade of eggplants is as soft as newborn hair; I run my hand along its contours, relishing the comforting feel. I search for anything soothing and warm to fight the ache in my heart and the ice fingers that have a strangle hold on my soul.

I extract myself from my daze and watch Dr. Thede reach toward a pile of folders filled with paper from the table in front of her. I swallow hard against the knot of anxiety rising up in my throat, while Steve leans forward from the sofa as though ready to leap from its grasp at any moment, his primal instinct of fight or flight ready to explode. She looks at us across the arrangement of salmon-colored silk lilies and the arc of magazines splayed across the table. "Let's discuss the findings of Kamy's testing, okay?"

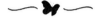

Ten weeks ago, Steve and I sat in this very spot. Ten weeks ago, we met Dr. Thede for the first time. Ten weeks ago, we embarked on a journey, a quest of discovery, not of treasure or unknown locations, but the answer to what plagued our daughter. We came to her doorstep, naive and unsure, sent by our family therapist who ran out of answers to explain Kamy's condition. This was not new to us; we encountered several professionals in the psychiatric field who considered our oldest daughter an enigma. We shuffled from therapist to therapist who dug into their bag of tricks to try to define the source of the demons that infested her mind. We ran the gambit of diagnoses until it came to a point that she exhibited the signs of so many mental disorders that not one single illness encompassed her. Beyond the scope of explanation with simple terms, our therapist advised that we have Kamy undergo intensive psychological testing in order to provide a definitive diagnosis. We came in search of answers; ask and you shall receive.

Our first appointment with Dr. Thede was a three-hour session that Steve and I attended without Kamy. It was rare for us to have any time to ourselves considering our situation, so we relished the car ride to the appointment. We rode in silence, lost in the tranquility of those fifteen minutes. Our lives no longer belonged to us, but to Kamy's illnesses. We abandoned normal long ago in favor of survival—our family outings, date nights, and quiet evenings replaced with doctor's appointments, psychotic rages, and battling unforeseen demons that lurked deep within her mind.

We had no idea what to expect. Three hours seemed like an eternity. We sat in her office holding hands in an act of comfort and solidarity against whatever we faced. We began the session with an explanation of the testing procedure. She walked us through step by step, providing us instructions on how to disassemble your child. "First, I meet with the two of you for six sessions, each about two hours long. We go over Kamy's history, beginning from birth. Then, there are several diagnostic questionnaires that you answer. Finally, I meet with Kamy for three sessions and walk her through a series of exams. I won't push her too much so as not to upset her. I work within her capabilities, okay?" She looked at us, a smile pulled at the corners of her mouth. Was she laughing? I wasn't sure. Perhaps she found joy destroying a family. I cleared such hostile thoughts from my mind, placed there by my maternal defense mechanism.

"How long before we know the results of the testing?" I asked as I fiddled with the zipper on my sweatshirt.

"About a month after we complete all of the testing, you come back in and we go over the results and measure out the appropriate steps to take from there," she said as she thumbed through her appointment book on her desk. "Let's see, we can get started with some of your part today and then we can schedule the rest of our appointments. Does that sound good to you?" I wanted to say, *No it doesn't sound good, none of this sounds good. I should be planning sleepovers, signing her up for soccer, taking her and her sister to movies and the zoo. Instead, I'm here.* Instead, I nodded and settled in for the afternoon.

Over the course of the next six weeks, Steve and I traveled across town to endure grueling interview sessions and daunting psychiatric questionnaires that rocked the very foundation of our parenting. We scrolled through endless questions that asked every awful reality a parent endures with a mentally ill child:

On a scale from one to five, one being never, and five being always, answer the following questions:

> *Does your child hear voices?*
> *Does your child exhibit extreme anger?*
> *Does your child break things?*
> *Does your child act inappropriate in public?*
> *Is your child physically aggressive?*
> *Does your child exhibit psychosomatic symptoms?*
> *Does your child suffer from delusions?*
> *Is your child subject to violent mood swings?*
> *Does your child engage in obsessive behaviors like washing hands repeatedly or constantly turning on and off the lights?*
> *Does your child have to follow a set routine?*
> *Is your child fearful of change?*

The questions were endless as they spilled down the page, each one documenting our lives over the past several years. I ticked off boxes to answer each: five, five, five, five, five in a continuous pattern. Steve let out a nervous laugh, running his fingers through his dark blond hair. "Has somebody been spying on us? They seem to know everything about our family." I looked at him. A light sheen of sweat settled upon his forehead; he sat hunched over his knees in the chair as though about to vomit.

"Hang in there, we're almost done," I tried to reassure him, but inside, my own mind was reeling. What did this mean? How was it that Kamy's behavior existed on the most extreme level to each question I answered? What kind of child lived in my home? What kind of madness had I bred inside my womb? Fear settled down next to me, amused as it watched me squirm.

It wasn't that any of these behaviors came as a shock to us; we endured Kamy's problems for over seven years. At first we resisted therapy and drug intervention; we thought we could handle the situation on our own—keep it in the family. As time went on, however, and she continued to descend into chasms of no retreat, we sought medical help. Four therapists and doctors and several medications later, we sat, a ream of paper in front of us prophesying our daughter's future.

After we waded through the questionnaires, we prepared ourselves for the interview sessions. We spent hours with her, recounting every detail of Kamy's life, from her inception up to the present. We unearthed every behavior and quirk she exhibited as a baby and toddler that could provide insight into her problems today, the fact that she didn't have any friends, her need for constant attention, eating problems as a baby. Any morsel of information I dredged up from my memory offered insight for the evaluation.

"Did Kamy have a lot of nightmares as a child?" she asked during one of the sessions.

"Yes, she did," I said, "she thought that people lived in the paint on her bedroom walls. She said they crawled across the walls at night. I sponge painted her room purple when she was two." Dr. Thede jotted something down in her notes. *Oh-oh*, I thought, *that can't be good.* Had my untrained artistry somehow triggered a mental break in my child?

"Did you breast-feed Kamy?" Her eyes bored into mine.

"No," my pulse pounded out a tympani in my head, "I bottle-fed both of my daughters."

"I see." Again, she continued with the incessant scribbling.

What the hell is she writing down? I wondered. Was my selfishness the reason I sat here today? Was I an inadequate mother? Guilt overwhelmed me. Was I to blame for my daughter's state? I knew guilt well; it set up shop in my soul from the time Kamy first started exhibiting signs of mental illness. Guilt and I were close friends.

Steve and I survived our part of Kamy's testing; now it was her turn. Kamy is suspicious of new people and the prospect of getting her to open up to another doctor caused anxiety for Steve and me. We knew that without her complete disclosure, Dr. Thede could not make a correct diagnosis. The first afternoon of her testing, we drove Kamy to Dr. Thede's office. She sat in the back seat, a sour look fixed on her face as she gazed out the window. Her hands clutched a stuffed horse and wolf; she whispered quietly to them as she stroked their fur matted by her obsessive touch. This sight might cause other parents to pause, given the fact that Kamy was eleven at the time. While most children her age abandon their interest in toys for more age-appropriate things like music, sports, and friends, Kamy remained trapped in early childhood. While her physical presence (her burgeoning figure and her expanding height) hinted toward the emergence of an adolescent girl, inside she remained the perpetual five-year-old, lost in fantasies of toys and games.

I looked back at her and tried to engage her blank stare. "You doing alright, Kam?" Blue eyes deep and endless as the sky looked back at me, void of any emotion. Jordan, seated next to her sister, quietly watched the scenery pass outside the car window. I pondered how a seven-year-old coped with living with a chronically ill sibling. I couldn't fathom the level of tolerance she possessed.

"I guess," she mumbled. "Why do I have to go?"

"So we can better understand your illnesses and know the best medicines and help to give you." *That's not going to fly*, I thought, *way too rational.*

"Why can't Ellie do that?" she asked, referring to her therapist.

"Dr. Thede is trained to do this. Don't worry, it's fine. Daddy and I are here with you, okay?" I tried to sound cheerful as I waited for her to erupt in a fury of screams and tears. Nothing. She turned back to her animals; I turned back to the front, isolated from her.

Dr. Thede was prepared for Kamy. She introduced herself to Kamy, who stood pressed against the wall. She knew not to touch Kamy, for any type of physical contact with another, even the slightest brush of her hand, causes her to react violently. She plied her with toys in her office and promises of the fun games they could play together. Kamy, resistant at first, ultimately gave way to the prospect of whiling away the afternoon engaged in her favorite activities. Steve, Jordan, and I settled ourselves into the waiting room for the two-hour wait. I wondered what magic occurred beyond the closed door, what incantations the good doctor could utter to extract the venom that poisons my daughter's mind. I glanced at Jordan as she sat drawing and coloring in her sketch pad, so happy and peaceful, nothing like her sister, who remains locked in her madness.

We accompanied Kamy to three more meetings with Dr. Thede. She ran Kamy through a battery of tests set to measure every aspect of her being, from her intelligence level, to her social skills, to her adaptability levels. For Kamy, it was a game. She did math problems, solved puzzles and riddles, acted out scenes with toys, unaware that with each choice she made, she further solidified her fate, saddled with the label of mentally ill forever. At the end of her last session, Dr. Thede emerged from her office, a look of triumph on her face. "We're finished!" she proclaimed. Kamy followed her from the room, a picture of a pencil-sketched horse in her hand.

"Look Mommy, I drew Dr. Thede a picture for her wall." I looked at the sketch. Kamy is a magnificent artist and her rendition of a young stallion rearing in the air was a remarkable likeness. Like other great artists who suffered from mental afflictions like Van Gogh, Picasso, and Pollack, Kamy finds escape in her art, a talent born from the chaos that lurks deep within her mind. Dr. Thede taped the picture up next to an inked caricature of a plump boy with a skeleton head and then turned to me.

"I'll go over everything myself and have my colleague concur with my findings before I write my final report. I'll call you when you can come in and find out the results." I thanked her and gathered up Jordan's belongings as Steve shepherded the girls out into the hallway. I bundled them up in their coats and followed Steve to our car. It was six o'clock; the haze from the late October evening dropped, cloaking us in the night.

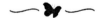

Now, ten weeks since that first day, we sit, anxious and scared, but of what—monsters, illness, ourselves, Kamy, our shame? Dr. Thede pulls out the papers from the folder and hands us an organized stack fastened together with a gold paper clip. She puts a pair of tortoiseshell rimmed glasses on and flips to the first page of her copy. "This is my official report, the one you use for all of Kamy's future treatment, as well as for your application for Social Security benefits for her. It contains everything you need with regard to her diagnoses." I notice the plural, not one but many. I shudder against the iced reality that blasts into my face.

For the next hour, Steve and I sit in silence as we listen to the doctor ramble on about the multitude of tests conducted and the findings. She explains raw scores and composite scores, scientific babble which falls on deaf ears; I want the brutal and naked truth without all of the psychoanalytical jargon that obscures the truth about Kamy. We reach the final page, the meat and potatoes of the report where everything is summarized with apathetic detail. I see the bold black letters that proclaim "Diagnoses" followed by a string of illnesses I am not soon to ever forget. They are staggering and severe. On this day, I learn my daughter's fate, and ultimately mine as well. On this day, the door closes forever on what small ray of hope to which I clung. I realize the cruel humor the universe employs as it randomly selects its prey. On this day, I weep for our loss. My daughter is no longer a person but a string of psychological maladies that rule her life; she is helpless against the frontal assault on her mind.

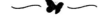

Confidential Neuropsychological Evaluation

Name of Patient: Kamryn Vought
Gender: Female
Testing Dates: 10/12/10–11/04/10
Age: 11

Assessment Methods:

Clinical Interview with Parents and
    Child
Mental Status Exam
Shipley 2
Wide Range Achievement Test
Gilliam Asperger Disorder scale
Autism Diagnostic Interview-Revised
Vineland II
Tree-in-a-Storm (Projective)

Trails A & B
Controlled Word Association
Token Test
Bender-Gestalt II
Child Bipolar Questionnaire
Autism Diagnostic Observation Sched-
    ule-Module 3
Child Behavioral Checklist

Presenting Problem:
Kamryn suffers
clinically significant behavioral issues of concern
beginning around the time she turned two:

failure to develop
        peer relationships
lack of spontaneously seeking

joy

lack of emotional
reciprocity inappropriate
comments and behaviors in public
        restricted

patterns of interest
resistance to change
in her routines or environment
and inflexible
        adherence to rituals.
These behaviors result in:
                clinically significant impairment
in Kamryn's social functioning
Kamryn also displays
periods during which she is   exceptional(ly)
irritable—moody
suffers
sleep disturbances and has explosive outbursts

occasionally sees or hears things
others do not
she bullies her younger sister
acts in an manner
            oppositional
                        toward her parents
has periods of high anxiety
during which she suffers gastrointestinal issues
is impulsive aggressive

although she never has spoken
suicide
parents report she lacks energy prefers

alone

can be
secretive
fearful
worrying,

cries more often

Collectively these symptoms and testing results support diagnoses:

296.7 Bipolar Disorder with Psychotic
Tendencies (auditory and visual hallucinations support this diagnosis)

299.80 Asperger's Syndrome

Other impairments unspecified

(As advised by *Diagnostic and Statistical Manual of Mental Disorders* when an individual meets criteria for a pervasive developmental disorder)
include Attention Deficit
Disorder and Mixed Receptive Expressive
Language Disorder
Consider these additional problem
areas as they may significantly impact Kamryn's
academic performance and occupational outlook

Prognosis: Poor
Recommendation:
Pray

Steve and I sit back. The report spills before us in a hideous stain. I clutch the side of the sofa. The velour no longer soothes me; it's cold and slick like a viper's side. I stop the tears. *I can't cry. I have to stay strong.* The room is silent; the only sound comes from the continuous gurgle of the fountain.

Steve lets out a pained sigh and clears his throat. "I know this is a lot to take in," Dr. Thede says. "Perhaps you need to digest this for a few days before we talk about treatment and Kamy's future outlook." Future? What kind of future waits for someone plagued by such misery? I look at her, angry and confused.

"What does this all mean?" I am not ignorant. Steve and I prepared for the worst case scenario when we began this process, but neither of us had any idea of how severe the outcome.

"Kamy will require support and care the rest of her life," Dr. Thede began, "she will most likely never hold a job or be able to live on her own. This is the reality people so burdened by their diseases face." She went on to describe the testing results: Kamy scored low on the living adaptability scale that measures her daily living, community, and domestic skills; Kamy scored low on the social integration and interpersonal relating scale; Kamy scored low on the receptive and expressive language scale; Kamy scored high on the maladaptive behavior index; Kamy scored high in oppositional defiant, aggressive, social deviant, rule-breaking, obsessive compulsive, and conduct problems. On and on and on she rambles off a list of Kamy's malformation, a description of a mind so twisted and confused that no soul could ever escape the labyrinth of the diseases. What amalgam of madness do we face?

Armed with our new knowledge and a heavy heart, we wander from the office dazed and confused by the mortar attack we survived. As I button up my coat, I remember the couple I watched leave only a short while before. What devastation had they endured? What news did they receive that forever shifted the balance of normalcy in their lives, just as it had ours? Mental illness destroys; there is no solution, no fix—no cure. It is the thief that robbed my daughter of her mind. It is the predator that secreted my child away into the umbra. It is the vacuum that leaves this mother's heart empty. It is goodbye.

The snow covers the hood of our car in a quilt. I listen to our shoes crunch in the fallen flakes beneath us. *Maybe tomorrow I'll let the girls play outside*, I think, *they love to play in the snow*. I can't wait to get home, to wrap my arms around Jordan and hold her close. I can't wait to see Kamy and tell her how much I love her; I can't hug or kiss her, but I love her all the same. I look at Steve and offer a weary smile. We share a quiet moment of understanding between us, a shared knowledge of the steep and winding road we face.

Steve backs the car out and takes a slow turn onto the road paved with diamond ice. I glance back at the building as it rises up against the night like the leviathan from the depths of the sea. Its hulking presence attempts to douse the filtered light. I won't let it. I hate that place. I hate this day. I love my daughter. God grant me serenity.

Snowfall

Snow descends.
Layers of silence
interspersed
with winter's melancholy
in still air, softens
the squeak of boots coming
up the road. Deepened still
with discontent, it tremors,
shatters the world
to pieces, deceptive
spheres that hide
their edges, etching
their face onto
window, wall, door.
It doesn't linger long;
it dwindles, returns
to clouds gray
as sifted ashes.

Some, upon finding a butterfly with crinkled or deformed wings, choose to intervene instead of ending its life. The debilitated creatures cannot survive on their own. They require constant care. If this is the choice made, provide it a safe area with plenty of space to move about, something to which it can cling. If the butterfly falls to the ground and fights to turn over, give it something to stabilize itself and pull itself upright again. Try other means of intervention to help its wings mend; if nothing can be done to straighten them or cure the disease that ails them, provide the butterfly with a home, food, and care for the rest of its life.

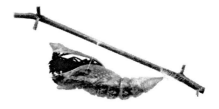

II.

A mother's heart is always with her children.

—*Proverb*

Mornings in our home do not run like clockwork. I roll everyone out of bed to start the day. Jordan greets me with a lazy smile and a wave from her bed. "Good morning, Bean. How did you sleep?"

"I slept good," she murmurs, grabbing my hand and kissing it. "How did you sleep?"

"Okay."

"You can always sleep down here with me. I'll let you sleep with Beast," she says, handing me her favorite stuffed polar bear.

I pat Beast on the head, "Thanks, but you keep her. I'm fine." I kiss her tousled blond hair and leave her room, which is adorned with Barbie dolls, princess wallpaper, and Eiffel Tower posters—the ideal ten-year-old girl's domain.

Waking Kamy is not so easy. She slips into a drug-induced coma every evening from which thundering elephants or tornadoes could not arouse. Her medication eases her into sleep, shutting down her hypervigilant brain that kept her awake at night when she first fell ill. Steve and I slept on a pull-out bed next to her room for seven months while enduring her nightly panic attacks. She refused sleep; sleep equated death. Fear consumed her at night, an agitation so extreme she vomited from fright, collapsing into slumber from exhaustion afterward. Now, powerful psychotropic medications offer her repose from her raving mind. Her medication-induced dreams provide topics for some fantastic and frightening dinnertime conversations: driving race cars with her stuffed penguin, a bright blue mansion in which we all live, a Yeti that plucks her sister from the bathtub and eats her.

I open the slats of her blind; sun streams in across her bed bursting with blankets and stuffed animals. Her room is filled with superhero paraphernalia: Spiderman posters; Marvel action figure; tiny toy weapons; sketches of her favorite hero, Captain America; all objects that enhance her illusions of reality. "Kamy, time to get up. Let's get going." After several minutes, she stirs in the bed.

Upon rising, she asks me, "Should I go to the bathroom now?"

"Yes, you need to go before breakfast." This is not an unusual question for her. She does not understand any type of cues from herself or others, making it impossible for her to decipher appropriate and normal behavior. When is the right time to use the restroom? For Kamy, it is whenever I tell her.

Kamy has one chore she must perform every day: making her bed. It takes up to half an hour for her to pull up her covers and place her stuffed animals on her bed. Most days, she ends up screaming if her comforter does not pull up with ease or if her blankets do not fold as easily as she desires. She sleeps with a congregation of nearly four dozen stuffed animals that she arranges in the same configuration in her bed every night, along with a collection of hats that she places in a specific order at the bottom of her bed. She prepares her bed the same way each night. If one object varies even the slightest from its standard assignment, she refuses to go to sleep, a symptom of her Asperger's syndrome and her obsessive compulsive disorder. As a result, the reconstruction of her sleep space for the day takes an eternity. Bed Making 101 for the mother of a mentally ill child: patience is your only virtue.

We share breakfast together every morning, a gathering for moral support and communion as we face each challenging day. I prepare Kamy's morning medication and measure out specific amounts of cereal and juice for her meal. I manage her food intake; if not, I elevate her risk of suffering from diabetes, heart disease, or liver malfunction, side effects of the potent chemicals coursing through her body. Kamy loves to eat, but she has no concept of regulation or self-control, no internal voice telling her no, issues that people with bipolar disorder on the severe end of the spectrum, like Kamy, battle every day. She tells me, "I could eat until I explode," as she inhales her meal with fervor, groaning and smacking with delight while the rest of us sit bemused by her obvious pleasure. Such behaviors have the potential to flourish into other addictions: drugs, alcohol, sex. For now, I am thankful that putting her through a Captain Crunch detox is my only worry.

It is a good morning today; Kamy appears in better spirits. I serve as her mood barometer as she has no self-awareness or ability to recognize her own emotions. Her illnesses rob her of such essential skills. She relies upon me to provide her with what her fractured mind cannot, an external compass to point her in the right direction. The day we encounter depends on her mood that morning. Some days she stares right through me, vacant eyes distant and unaware of her surroundings. Other days, I spot the rage building behind her gaze, her face pinched in a grimace. Nothing gets accomplished on those days; those are black days.

After breakfast, I hurry everyone along to their prospective tasks: school for the girls and work for Steve. Steve works from home now. He was a deputy sheriff and a criminal investigator in a previous life, before the onset of Kamy's illnesses. He owns and operates an investigation and genealogy business now, contracting with local companies and attorneys who value his services. We made the decision that his previous work added too much stress to our lives when coupled with Kamy's issues. Working from home allows him to help with Kamy's care, a sacrifice of his independence, but one he takes in stride. The years of stress pepper his dark blond hair with gray and steal the impish gleam from his eyes, the same faded blue as Kamryn's.

Kamy's illnesses forced our relationship into a new genre of marriage. Once we were idealistic lovers and companions. Now we exist as allies, fighting for our daughter and the sanctity of our family. High fives now replace kisses; a comforting hand on the shoulder supplants a passionate embrace. We are not alone in our evolution. Any parent who lives with a child who is mentally ill undergoes a major overhaul of his or her assumed normal existence. Blogs and websites dedicated to supporting families of the mentally ill are choked with personal accounts of parents reaching out to find common ground with others who suffer their same fate. Many couples do not survive the stress of mental illness, their marriages falling to waste.

There were times when the resentment and tension between us stole the air from the room, choking me like thick cotton wedged into my chest. We fought about everything, knock down drag outs about the most ridiculous things: forgetting to empty the trash, what to have for dinner, taking too long to run an errand. Outward hostilities hid our inner grief; we both suffered from the loss of our daughter and the mental and physical drain caring for a chronically ill child has on the spirit. I screamed at him; he would take off in our only car for hours on end. I called him a horrible father; he told me I was to blame for Kamy's condition.

Many nights, I slept on the floor in our study, wrapped in a blanket and my sorrow, silent tears saturating the pillow beneath my head. We teetered each day closer to the edge of divorce, both threatening to leave the other, yet both petrified to face life alone. Somehow, either through grace or exhaustion, we remained true to each other, even still today. I wake up every morning next to him, thankful to have a partner in life. Despite all the adversity we face, we persevere, vowing to each other daily to remain strong and steadfast, for our love, for our marriage, and for our family.

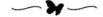

I Love You More Today

It's possible to wake up
and not recognize
your surroundings. How passionate
our existence, full of spirit
and love. I liked the part
I played, my performance
brilliant, my fantasy clever.
I memorized your shape.
The sun sank in the sky; shadows
lengthened and grew, eclipsing light.

My loving weakness screams
loud and long. I threw a chair
at your shattered reflection.
Resent climbs into bed
between us. Awareness grows
that we are no longer friends,
only acquaintances; recognize
we reached the end. Keep
our secret silent, liquefy the children
with our explosions. Reach into
your cache of black words, toss them
like Chinese stars at my heart.
Celebrate the futility
of our determination like an ant
crawling up an oiled mountain.

Order has no place
in our lives. Do you remember
the two of us, before pleasure incited
the embryo hurling
a computer in your direction?
Blue eyes, cloned
from your atoms colliding
with mine, brim with fear
and hate. Famous house
where the abomination
of our love resides. Police
come to our earmarked location.
One sits at the kitchen
table, gun dug into his bloated
side; I recognize him

from last time we unraveled.
How did our love create
this child? There is no way

to prepare, the future a promise
with no guarantees, the past
a mirror for wishful thinking.
We find and lose
each other. Love is a union
of spirit and being.
Outside, people come
home, lift their windows
to a life curling into sky.
In here, we surrender
to our calling. I love you
more today.

Recognition and respect for the other person's feelings is vital in order to preserve a relationship that endures endless stress. A healthy and twisted sense of humor does not hurt either. Who else can laugh with you about the most obscene things your child does while enduring the sorrow, surrealism, and magnitude of the situation: Kamy clogging the toilet with an excess of toilet paper from wiping a dozen times, watching the same movie every night for three months straight, drawing pictures of the movie and recording the soundtrack on her iPod from YouTube postings so as to immerse herself in it even more, peeling the paint off her bedroom wall, or collecting clusters of fuzz and used Kleenex in her nightstand drawer. We often kid that the only way anyone would believe our lives is if we documented it with video evidence. If we did not fall into each other's arms laughing we might, too, go mad. We live crazy; without acknowledging such, everything else fails.

Every day I must tell Kamy what to wear, not by choice, but by necessity: "Mommy, what should I wear today, short sleeve or long sleeve? Should I wear pants? Can you help me put on my bra? Which shirt should I wear? Will this one be okay?" I listen to the same mantra every morning, a part of her ritualized routine. If it's snowing, Kamy wonders if she can wear shorts or her bathing suit. If it's eighty degrees, she wants to wear her snow hat and fleece-lined boots. Weather has no effect on her delirium. We live in opposite world, where the sky is green and the grass grows blue. I always remind myself that her mature physical appearance does not reflect the child within, lost and confused, trapped in a perpetual haze.

Nonsense and repetition, though infuriating to me, prove vital for her skewed sense of sanity. If I find comfort in one thing, however, it is the fact that Kamy sees herself in a positive light, unmoved by her debilitating diseases. As God crippled her mind, he also blessed her with ignorant bliss. Kamy relishes her condition, finding nothing wrong with her mental illness. She understands her conditions, but in her mind, she is as healthy and functional as the rest of us, unmoved by the fact that her brain inhibits her abilities to operate normally. After she suffers a bout of uncontrollable anger, she tells me, "It's just because I am bipolar," dismissing any other explanation as false. If I point out her fixations, her obsessing to the point of neurosis, she states with satisfaction, "It's just my Asperger's," brushing aside the notion that anything is out of the ordinary. Kamy does not deny her illnesses but immerses herself in them. In her mind, we are flawed, not her—blind to how others perceive her. I welcome such unawareness of herself and her surroundings in this case, for it protects her from the biases and judgment passed by a world cruel and insular to the mentally ill.

I walk Kamy through her morning personal hygiene routine every day. Asperger's syndrome inhibits her ability to care for herself in the same manner as her peers. She could burn down the house trying to cook her meals, spend her income on video games instead of food, attack a neighbor because he spoke to her during a manic phase, go weeks without washing her hair, or sink into a delusional nightmare where voices speak to her from the television because she forgot to take her medication. Kamy is my responsibility for the rest of my life. I am forever her custodian; she is incapable of living unassisted. I never imagined caring for my children beyond their adolescence. I hoped they would grow to lead their own lives, independent from me.

This is one of those mornings when I imagine myself far away from this life. Sometimes I fantasize about getting into a car and just driving away, never seen or heard from again, the monotony of my life with her gone. I ponder the condition of my life without children: quiet, peaceful, serene. Not all days, but some. I imagine myself a philanthropist donating my earnings to the Humane Society; a writer crafting the most remarkable works of literature in an isolated cabin on a horse ranch on the western slope of Colorado; a humanitarian visiting women in Africa who are survivors of genital mutilation, infusing them with courage and strength; an environmentalist tossed about in the Antarctic Sea aboard a small raft squaring off with a whaling vessel; a world traveler sipping Bordeaux in Nice one day, only to sample Baklava in Crete the next. I am every woman, fulfilling every wish, dream, and desire. I have no one dependent upon me, no one demanding my attention twenty-four hours a day; I am myself, my own woman, free once more.

Farewell Mon Amie

I'm sorry, dear
friend, for my apathy
and indiscretion. Shadows
crawl from my mouth, eclipse
your smile.Wet air hangs
limp as acetone laundry
left to spoil in the sun.
You ran when butterflies
fled in drunken flight
from my cruelty.

I apologize for my neglect.
I forgot the garden
in your absence.Where
you blossomed, weeds
infest, wrap their spindles
around my vacant home.
Laughter twisted from you
like a ribbon.You watched
the children play hide
and go seek, camouflaged
by clouds. I made you
come inside my bitterness.

I caged your joy.
You lie alone in your
limestone cell while I cry
crocodile tears. I drank wine
as your gashes festered. My
edge sank into your chest. Joy
spilled. I consumed the remains.

Forgive my misguided
hand. I touch your face
upon my looking glass.
It peers out, mirrored eyes
exact. I lie in our bed,
lonely for your company.
Papayas and cocoa butter
rest on your pillow. I sent you
far away where the rooster
crows Hosanna, praise be.

I betrayed you, guided you
where God extinguished
the stars. Please return
to my reflection. I am an aching
memory without you.

I clear my head from my daydreams and return to my daily task, reminding Kamy to brush her teeth. She sometimes brushes her teeth so hard and long that her gums bleed. If she finds any flaw or spec of foreign substance, she flies into a panic, yet she refuses to visit the dentist for fear of anyone touching her. She is terrified of germs or illness of any kind. I cannot count how many times I convinced her that she does not have a brain tumor because she forgets something, or heart disease because she suffers a slight twinge in her chest. How often have I calmed the numerous panic attacks she suffers because she thinks she feels her throat closing. She washes her hands at least a dozen times each day in an effort to eradicate invisible enemies from her chapped and cracked skin, demanding that we all do the same. She times on her watch how long to wash them, the same amount each time, exactly three pumps of soap in her hands, demented in her exactness.

She ascends the stairs this morning, after cleaning her teeth, upset because Jordan told her to get out of her room. Kamy plays aggressively. She cannot regulate her exuberance just as she cannot control her anger, and in her attempt to "play," she broke Jordan's stained glass night-light fashioned in the shape of a horse's head. "I'm never playing with her again," Kamy states in a defiant tone, a pout affixed in place, clutching her bundle of stuffed animals she carries everywhere. "I didn't mean to break the light." Although Kamy is fourteen biologically, her stunted emotional and social development leaves me with a four-year-old who outweighs me by twenty pounds and is only one inch shorter than me. When I discipline or try to reason with her, I revert to my early days of motherhood, parenting a child trapped in her immaturity.

I fix Kamy's hair every day as part of her morning schedule. She arrives in my bathroom with a ratted mess of tangles that she neglected to brush herself downstairs. As I smooth down her long honeyed hair, I contemplate taking the scissors and cutting it all off, making my life easier in the end. I know that is not a possibility; Kamy won't let anyone cut her hair. Haircuts frighten her. She allows me to trim only a small amount off the ends now and again. I braid her hair every day. Pleased with the plait fashioned with my skilled hand, I cringe as she shoves a Yankees hat atop her head. She wears a hat every day, but not because of any aesthetic reason. In her tortured mind, hats protect her; she wears them for survival. She refuses to leave it off, except at night. She even wears one under her bike helmet.

As a result, the helmet sits atop her head like a mushroom, pushed up from the extra bulk of her hat. I have not seen my daughter without a baseball cap on her head in years. I reminisce about times long ago when I used to style her hair, placing tiny barrettes or clips in her soft golden hair, her doll face framed with delicate curls. Those days do not seem real anymore, a life someone else led—alive only in my memories.

Jordan comes prancing into the bathroom after Kamy, dressed in her best attire, a red and black sweater dress with black leggings and a matching scarf, a rhinestone headband atop her head, gold hair shining. She exists as Kamryn's antonym, her sister's contradiction: happy, carefree, sweet, and kind. She has endured more in her ten years than most encounter during their entire life. Her sister hits her, screams obscenities at her, threatens to kill her, and tells her that she hates her, all on a regular basis. Jordan watched while Steve put Kamy into a police hold after she tried to stab him with a pen. She comforted me after Kamy kicked me in the face, angry that I sent her to her room. She greets me every morning with a beautiful smile that makes me remember why I became a mother.

The compassion she harbors within her amazes me, always forgiving, always accepting of a sister who causes so much pain. She never complains, always focused on the positive aspects of life, planning her future amidst the ruins of

Kamy's: "When I get older, I want to be a fashion designer and live in Paris. When you come to my house, I'm going to make my famous pasta salad. I'm going to have a Persian cat and two Bichon Frise and maybe a parakeet. I'm going to grow my own vegetables. Maybe I will be a veterinarian too." Jordan's dreams and ideals only illuminate Kamy's lack thereof; Kamy's dream in life, as she loves to tell me time and again, is to "live on our front porch." Jordan's light radiates through the shadows that threaten to consume our family, a beacon in a dark and violent storm. She has more strength than I can comprehend, exiled from her childhood by her sister's diseases.

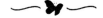

My Bean: For Jordan

catch a fistful of sun and name it
tie love like a string around my finger
record a chickadee's laughter
drink from a spring spouting nectar
gaze into God's eyes
I find you

For a few moments, after I braid Kamy's hair, I close myself into my bathroom, entombed in its cubical space. I do not have a large and luxurious bathroom, but a simple room that serves to function, not indulge. I turn on the blow dryer and lay it on the counter, the constant hum drowning all noise outside. I create a porcelain oasis free from the tempest lurking just beyond the door. Here I sit and contemplate my life. How did I get here? Will this ever end? I gather strength in my small space. I have no choice. I am the core of our structure—the family stone. I cannot fall to depression's advances. I refuse. If I keep myself moving it cannot catch me. I lie if I say that days do not exist, Kamy at her worst, stuck in a manic phase, when the self-pity creeps in—my "why me" phase—but I remain vigilant against the temptation to fall into its trap, forever lost in my sorrow. Who will care for Kamy if I fall?

Admittedly, Kamy's illnesses devastate me. I buried all of the images I bore in my mind of Kamy's future: proms, graduations, soccer games, dance recitals, weddings. New images surfaced, disturbing visions fueled by the negative perceptions of the mentally ill: Kamy the drug addict, the prisoner, the vagabond, the dropout, the criminal—the lunatic. Doctors and therapists prepared us for the devastation. We face a life-long battle with her diseased mind. Things will never be easy for us, and even more difficult for Kamy. Her illnesses paint a mark upon her chest, branding her "different," an anomaly of nature.

Our world, as progressive as it seems upon the surface, remains trapped in the dark ages with regard to mental health acceptance and support. After all, only a few decades ago society locked away the mentally ill, left to dwell in squalor, sitting in their own waste while medical staff ill-equipped to handle their complex illnesses employed treatments of the most horrific nature. History reveals that the mentally handicapped were the first "euthanasia killings" the Nazis organized, a sort of practice run for their future systematic execution of the Jews. They never knew the comfort of a mother's embrace, the warmth of the sun on their faces as they strolled about a lake, the pleasure of laughter and joy. Services today still lack, and the perception of those afflicted with mental illness is skewed. Our daughter exists on the fray, residing on the cusp of normalcy, denied access because of her altered state. She is an outsider gazing into our right-minded world.

Such a prognosis is difficult to accept. I diverged down a path of self-pity, wallowing in grief over the loss of my "normal" child. I felt ashamed of her, embarrassed by her oddities that made her stand out from mainstream society. I hated going shopping with her, guiding her around the store by the arm because she lacked the insight on how to effectively handle a social situation. I despised the stares and whispers from others when they witnessed one of her frequent outbursts. I stayed at home with her, sending my husband on errands so as to avoid the public spectacles. I refused to see her as mentally ill, instead blaming her problems on my lack of parenting skills. I believed my inadequacies as a mother led to her current state. I refused to acknowledge the signs of her diseased brain. Instead, I focused my efforts on how to cure her. If this situation was indeed a result of me stumbling down the road of motherhood, then by God, I would fix it. I broke her; I could restore her.

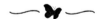

Don't Tell Me

Pay no attention
to words they say:

She has a curious way about her.
She's not like us, try as she might.
Mothers deserve to choose what they give birth to.

Shut up! Shut up!

She doesn't mean to be cruel.
She does what she wants.
She fears turning into shadows.
She thinks she can't enter Heaven.
She presses against me, demanding more.
She has her own song.

God looked right through her,
transparent as invisible glass.
He forgot to keep track that day.

I read articles on nutrition and its impact upon behavior, learned the vitamin supplements that impacted a child's social and mental development, researched every holistic treatment for her psychosomatic digestive issues. I purchased supplements and probiotics, cut her sugar intake, implemented tough love techniques, threatened her, yelled at her, and cried myself to sleep every night, frustrated and exhausted by another day with no progress. Each day I awakened rejuvenated, certain that the morning brought a new beginning; soon my hope and denial turned to defeat, sorrow—resolve.

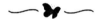

My reckoning came one evening when I found myself engaged in yet another battle with Kamy. Before we sought help through therapy, Steve and I tried our best to self-diagnose her problems. Each time she had an incident, I spent the next several hours trying to unlock the mystery surrounding her behavior, certain if I knew what held the answer to her cryptic mind, I could remedy the situation.

On this particular night, Kamy beckoned us to her room yet again well after midnight, fearing carbon monoxide poisoning. Convinced that the heating vents pumped poisonous fumes into her bedroom, she refused to go to sleep, hysterical over the prospect. "Kamy, you're keeping everyone up. You either go to bed or we're going to have problems," I yelled at her, frustrated over finding myself in the same predicament yet again.

"I can't!" she wailed. "My chest feels tight and I can't breathe!"

"That's because you're having a panic attack!"

"There's something wrong with me."

I exploded. "Enough! If you have something wrong, then I'll take you to the hospital!"

Steve pulled her from her bed. She fell to the ground, kicking and screaming, "Nooo! I don't want anyone else taking care of me! They're stupid! They don't know about me!"

I grabbed a sweatshirt and her Denver Bronco slippers from her closet. "Put these on," I demanded. She kicked at me, sweeping my leg like a soccer player and knocking me to the ground. As I tried to right myself, her foot made contact with the side of my face, a direct blow.

I pulled her up from the floor, infuriated by the physical assault. I pushed her upstairs and out into the garage. Steve and Jordan, awakened from her sleep by the commotion, trailed behind us. "Get in the car!" I screamed, not at all pleased with my behavior but driven by my principles to teach her a lesson. "Let the doctors at the hospital take care of you. I'm done!"

"No, Mommy, no!" she pleaded as she climbed into the backseat of our Xterra. I jumped into the driver's seat and fired up the ignition. I slammed the car into reverse and flew out of the garage.

"Janna, careful!" Steve yelled at me from the garage. I made out his silhouette in the low light cast from the single bulb protruding from the ceiling. My little Bean stood next to him in her nightgown—crying. My breath hitched; tears burned the corners of my eyes. I couldn't falter. I backed down the drive and headed into the night; the shadows consumed us.

I headed in the direction of the hospital, rambling off my doctrine of rules and appropriate behavior to Kamryn. "You can tell the doctors at the hospital that you're dying. You disrupt our home on a continual basis. I can't do this anymore. Let them figure out what is wrong and how to help you because you don't listen to me."

"I'm sorry, Mommy, please don't make me go!" I knew I wasn't taking her to the hospital, but I thought the fear of going would spur her to change her ways, back before I knew she has no control over her mind, let alone her behavior, back before she received her official diagnoses, back when I still held hope for a miracle. I rounded a corner, preparing to travel back toward our house, past a 7-Eleven and a gas station. As the car slowed, Kamy opened her door and jumped out of the car. I panicked; I could not believe what just happened. I saw her in the rearview mirror, illuminated by a lone streetlight, standing outside of an office building. I stopped in the middle of the road and threw the car in reverse, turning into the parking lot of the abandoned building. I didn't see her anywhere. I jumped out of the car, screaming her name into the darkness.

"Kamy! Kamy, where are you?" No answer. The fluorescent light from the 7-Eleven across the street lit the parking lot enough to where I could see her if she was still there; not a shadow stirred.

I jumped back in the Xterra and flew out of the parking lot. I circled the block, certain I would see her walking in her Bronco slippers. I rolled my window down, yelling for her out of the window. I circled the block three times in desperation before I allowed myself to acknowledge her absence. Only two minutes from our house by car, I drove home, hoping to find her waiting for me. "Please, God, please, God, please!" I cried, tears running, "I'm so sorry! Please forgive me, just bring her back to me!"

As I drove for those brief seconds, I envisioned every horrible scenario imaginable: a sexual predator stealing her away into the night, getting hit by a car whose driver couldn't see her cross the street in her dark blue hoodie, calling the police and filing a missing person's report, explaining to them how I tried to manipulate her behavior by taking her to a bogus hospital admittance. I pulled into our driveway and ran inside the house. Steve and Jordan sat in our bed, waiting for our return.

"She's gone!" I blurted. "She jumped out of the car when I turned the corner!" Steve leapt from the bed.

"Jesus, Janna!" he yelled as he headed for the car. I picked up Jordan and ran after him. I strapped her into the backseat and climbed in the front next to Steve. We took off. I directed him to the location where she jumped from the car, but there still was no sign of her. Steve pulled into the parking lot of the 7-Eleven across the street. "Wait here. I'm going to see if she came in here or if they saw anything." I gnawed on my thumbnail, peering out the window into the pitch in hopes of spotting her small frame part the darkness.

"Will we find Kiki?" a voice said from the backseat. I turned to look at Jordan, pressed against the doorframe, huddled beneath the coat I wrapped her in before we left.

"We'll find her, Bean, don't worry." I reached back and grabbed her hand, the smooth skin warm against my frigid grasp. A brush of cold air swept into the car from the driver's side door.

Steve folded into the seat. "She didn't go in and they don't remember seeing her either."

"Now what?" My voice crumbled under the stress of the moment.

"We need to go home and contact the police." He sighed and started the car. Fear took hold of me on the short drive home. It stroked my throbbing head, clasped its strong arms around my chest; it refused to let go.

We rode in silence; no one dared speak her name. As we turned into our driveway, the headlights cast a beacon of light across our front porch. There, perched on the top step in her Bronco slippers crusted in road grime, sat Kamy. I scrambled out of the car, sprinted across the grass and hurdled the first two steps, resting beside her. "Kamy, we looked everywhere for you! Where have you been?"

"I walked home down Poinsettia," she said, pointing to the street that ran adjacent to ours, one we neglected to travel during our search. "I ruined my slippers." She appeared unfazed by the incident, unlike the rest of us.

"Kamy, don't you ever do anything like that again. Do you understand me? You could hurt yourself or get lost." I wanted to hug her, to hold her against my breast, this daughter of my flesh and bone, and never let her go, but I couldn't. She wouldn't allow it. Underneath my calm demeanor, my heart soared. Never was I more thankful than in that moment, more certain than ever of my need to seek help for my daughter. This situation ballooned far beyond my control. I needed to intervene, before I lost her forever.

She stood up and smiled. "Okay, Mommy. I'm sorry I ran away, but I didn't want stupid doctors and nurses taking care of me. I don't trust anyone but you."

"Let's get you and Jordan to bed." We walked side by side into the house, so close in proximity but miles away from each other. I never fathomed a motherhood such as this, never comprehended the role God destined me to play in Kamy's life. I knew, however, that I no longer could turn away from the truth. I could no longer hide behind my anger and resentment. Reality demanded my full attention.

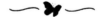

When I gave birth to my daughters, I celebrated the notion that God granted me the opportunity to raise the perfect mixture of Gloria Steinem, Mother Teresa, and Hilary Clinton: strong, independent women who would lead rich, productive, socially-redeeming, and successful lives. This was a tall order for anyone to fulfill, no doubt; I knew my expectations exceeded the probability of all of these dreams actually coming to fruition, but I felt if I aimed high, I could succeed in fulfilling at least some of them through the strong upbringing of my daughters. Now, I stood looking at what remained of my dreams—crumbled ruins at my feet. The prodigal phrase of Robert Frost echoed in my head: "Two roads diverged in a yellow wood, and sorry I could not travel both." I knew I had a choice to make, one that redefined not only my existence, but that of Kamy and our entire family as well. Kamy continued to spiral down into her illnesses while I busied myself concocting miracle cures in vain. How was I helping to improve her life by hiding in my own self-pity and denial? Would I turn away from my daughter, deny her authentic self, or embrace this experience and celebrate her life in its altered form?

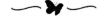

Into this World I Brought a Child

Into this world I brought a child,
flesh and bones of my own
creation. Spin the earth
to find another like her.

Molecules unravel promises
like a ball of twine, careening
through bramble gardens
until nothing remains.

Snags, twists, and tangles,
millions of miles of string determine
my daughter's destiny left to dangle
in the fury of her unclean mind.
I wish she had cancer, a limp,
something others see.
I tire of gawking, cry
tears I cannot swallow.

They cannot fix her; they try
and try. Time to give up
grieving for my daughter.
There's a girl I'll meet again

when generations end
and I receive Heaven.

I gaze into the mirror, stare into a face I no longer recognize. Dark circles rim my eyes; deep brown hair lies limp on my shoulders. *I need a haircut*, I say to myself, chuckling at the fact that I haven't had my hair styled since the onset of Kamy's illnesses. The extent of my hairstyling consists of trimming my ends while hunched over the bathroom sink. Of course, the elegant ponytail that dons my head every day is no worse for wear from my lack of a beauty regime. I exist as a quandary to the feminine ideal. I have not worn much beyond exercise clothes or t-shirts and jeans in years. Dresses flee in fear from my frame. Gathering my dark hair back into a ponytail and splashing water on my face, I remember where I am, what I must do—survive another day.

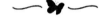

The Changeling

See what you suppose
is me. My beauty runs
from the crown of my head
deep underneath feet rooted
in deception. It's enough
to cause distraction.
My body, a cathedral
of matches, burns when my soul
retreats. At night I mix
almond milk and cement,
construct a mask that conceals
my shame, a human coat
of arms—thin and chipped armor.

On dark days I awaken, my heart
slumps against the wall. In me
are lives I do not recognize.
I loosen at the edges—
unwind. I am directionless,
a compass pointedWest.
Carry me back where
I began as a vision.

I sit on the edge of a tar
black hole. Life slips through
my fingers. Dreams
still throb within. The living
too tiny and lonesome
to recognize who they are.
I cannot work miracles; my water
remains clear—unrefined.
Pretend life something different
than my regrets. See me,
am I dead? Do I still
breathe? Then speak!

Chaos greets me the moment I exit the bathroom. "Mommy, can I hold the bird?" Kamy inquires, her eyes wide with anticipation as she sits next to a birdcage housing a gaily frocked parakeet. "Daddy told me no."

Steve chimes in, defending his actions. "I told her no because she needs to start her schoolwork." I try to remain calm, knowing the slightest elevation of my voice or wrong answer could send her into a rage.

"You have to start your lessons right now, but perhaps you can hold him later."

She looks disappointed, but recoverable: "Okay," she mumbles, stalking away.

Way to go! I commend myself; disaster averted. We homeschool the girls and getting Kamy to complete her work is not easy. I am the master negotiator, bartering trade deals diplomats envy. If I find a feasible offering—playing video games on the weekend, going for a bike ride after school, a new pack of trading cards—I serve it up in exchange for her compliance during school. It does not always work, but it is the best I can come up with in my illogical world.

I turn to Steve, exasperated by yet another conflict between him and Kamy. "You have to pick your battles. Some things aren't worth arguing with her." He looks at me, angry, defensive of his actions.

"I know, but I'm tired of her thinking she can do whatever she wants. It's the tail wagging the dog in this house." He strides away, mumbling to no one but himself: "Thanks, Kamy." I sigh, leaning against the kitchen counter. I referee my share of bouts between the two, always at each other for something. Steve doesn't know how to cope with or rectify his overwhelming emotions about Kamryn. "I don't like her, Janna. She ruins our lives," he often tells me after enduring another round with Kamy. I understand his frustration and pain. Who cannot feel despair when faced with a future saddled with her care? What happened to our best laid plans of family: vacations, holidays, and lifetime milestones shared with our loving brood?

During our therapy sessions, Steve sits quietly on the couch next to me, listening while I ramble on about our latest escapades with Kamy, steeped in his own misery. Instead of hugs, Kamy punches him in the stomach. Instead of sharing each other's company on an afternoon stroll to the park, Kamy attacks him on the side of the road, cars driving by filled with curious and shocked spectators who witness her assault on him. Instead of telling him she loves him, Kamy screams for him to get away. Kamy's illnesses strip him of the privilege of fathering in the way for which he longs—the doting daddy and the loving child. Instead, he finds himself in roles he never imagined: the warden, the bodyguard, the sentinel standing atop the watchtower, awaiting Kamy's next invasion.

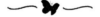

I go downstairs, but not before I assure Kamy that nothing is wrong with her, and descend into the basement to decompress. I don't take a nap on the couch or listen to Enya warble lyrics glazed in Celtic ethereality. I work out. I do not mean a Jane Fonda routine, pirouetting about the room in my leg warmers and matching leotard—I work. Seven days a week for an hour and a half, I brutalize my body, engage in physical exertion that ignites my body in tortured flames. The more difficult the exercise, the better; the heavier the weight, the more I push to lift it. If my shirt does not cling to my body drenched in sweat, I did not work hard enough. If I can talk at the end of my session, I failed. I am not a fitness freak, although I do enjoy the benefits of kicking my own ass every day. I exercise to release stress. I exert control over my body to compensate for the lack of rule in my life. I push my body to extreme limits to test my inner strength and will. With each drop of sweat purged from my skin, my spirit cleanses. I find focus, whether running for eight miles, enduring grueling circuit training sessions, or contorting my body into unnatural yoga positions. Exercise is my Valium. I take it every day.

When I am alone for this brief time, I search for God. He cannot penetrate the din of my life, but in the moments when my body surges with adrenaline, surrounded by silence, I clear my mind and create a pathway into my heart where he sits for a spell, old friends catching up on time lost. I am not a religious person, but I maintain a strong sense of spirit. In the beginning, I welcomed God in whenever he felt compelled to visit, my door always open to him. Then Kamy fell ill and guilt took over my space, saving no room for any other entity in my soul. I blamed myself for everything: the time I left her crying in her crib because I was too tired to pick her up, or the moments I abandoned her to the arms of another so I could have an afternoon free from a toddler clinging to my leg. Perhaps her infant immunizations infected her mind. I read about a possible link between vaccinations and autism and Asperger's syndrome. Could this be the reason for her condition? How do you choose: polio or debilitating developmental and mental illness? What twisted roulette wheel do I spin to decide my daughter's destiny? Did I stunt her social development because I chose to homeschool her? Is she better off without me? Did I have too much faith, or not enough? I scoured the recesses of my memory to come up with anything to explain why Kamryn wandered so far from home.

Faithful Masses

God, where are you? I search
alleyways and poppies
dancing, darkened highways
with one headlight, bedroom closets,
sandstone summits, my daughter's
smile. Children starve in fields filled
with grain. Abandoned babies cry.
Someone shot a boy
playing basketball. A man lost
his home. Why
didn't you come?

I hunt, toes unfurled
in tart brine crashing
upon a million grains of sand,
hermit crab expanding from his one
bedroom home. Do you swim
along shores carving lines
into tranquil blue, dodge
fish bones and ink plumes, hide
in ivory graveyards where elephants
remember love, along salted
breezes where albatross glide,
deep in pockets of pine
where sun never shines?

Others search for Heaven
in church rafters, eyes
turned toward clouds,
buoyant chapels dangling
in the sky. They rest
on sacred wood scratched
and worn, voices rejoicing,
swaying in black satin.
They follow without choice
like sunflowers follow light.
They gather, faithful masses,
and pray, pass the collection
plate, share unleavened bread
and sacramental wine,
trying just to kill some time.
I sit in silence as soft
as the mourning dove coo.
Where are you?

Undoubtedly, I was somehow to blame for my own loss; I brought this plague upon our family. I thought if I confessed the error of my ways, the doors of Heaven would spring open and return my girl. God hid her away from my sight, tucked away for safekeeping while I fumbled about in a strange and empty world. Only when I repented my sins of motherhood would God forgive me and set Kamryn free. What cruel tricks He plays on the vulnerable and weak. I toyed with the frayed edges of darkness. If God refused to return my child, then perhaps the devil could. I cared not about the sacrifice, willing to go to any ends to bring my daughter back in her absolute form.

The truth came swift and hard when Kamy's therapists and doctors solidified the grim future Kamy faced. She requires long-term care. Her risk of victimization, or worse, victimizing another, is extreme. Few support services exist that assist families with mentally ill children. Most operate in a reactive state, providing services only when the individual harms themselves or another or commits a crime. The only programs offering more than a sterile bed in an isolated and antiseptic location extend far beyond our financial capabilities. Although the federal government recognizes her as permanently disabled and pays her Social Security income, it does not begin to cover the monumental cost of her care. No knight rides in upon his steed, sword drawn, to fight for Kamy's life. It rests on our shoulders.

Her success as a human depends upon our ability to adapt our lives to her needs, and the more time I wallow in the mire of self-pity, the less I have to focus upon the care of my daughter and the preservation of my family. I swept guilt and self-loathing from my heart, parting ways with any blame. God tapped me on the shoulder: *Janna, do you remember me? I wept with you. We ran in fright, feet flying along the concrete, trying to escape memories of her. I picked you up when you fell. I am here with you—always.* I removed the bolts upon my door and let it swing wide once more, inviting God to walk with me, talk with me, steady my feet as I move forward in life, no matter what lies before me.

Mental illness is scary; it's frightening and cruel. It's also exceptional, exquisite—remarkable. I embark on this quest with trepidation; I spent so many years trying to pull her free from the hold mental illness had on her soul, but I now realize that in order for Kamy to thrive, I must embrace her mental illness, revel in it, experience her way of life. I tire of fighting the natural course of her existence; I want to be something more to my daughter than just her disciplinarian and caregiver; I want her to know that she is not alone.

Some people look at my acceptance of her illnesses as relinquishing control to the diseases, choosing to let me know of their own biases toward my decision: "If only you would try more," "You shouldn't homeschool her," "Maybe she just needs some friends," "Medication is not the answer," "Have you considered putting her in a special school?" Each comment fuels my desire more. I am weary of other's suggestions to pass her off to agencies eager to reap the financial benefits of her participation. I brought her into this world; she is my responsibility, through good and bad, thick and thin. This is the promise I made to her and to God.

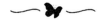

Letting Go

Her gray absence
hangs thick like January
clouds pregnant with snow.
I need a break
from endless sorrow.
Her obsolescence devastates
me, a dying star hurtled
toward Jupiter's blood
storm. A mother is created
to fight for her young.
I took in a stray dog
from the street, fed it meat,
cared for it, bathed it,
but its infection
was terminal.
I let go, surrendered
it to grace, cried
for it. My need
to pray for my mad
girl makes God
a necessity.

I return from my exercise sanctuary to face a heated battle over math problems and English lessons. "Kamy, we discussed proportions and ratios a dozen times already," Steve says. "I want you to try the problems on your own now."

"I hate math!" Kamy shrieks, slamming her fists down on her desk. "I'm not going to do this anymore!" She storms out of the room, pounding down the stairs to her room with so much force, the floor quakes beneath my feet.

"I explained it to her so many times. I don't know what else to do."

"It's difficult, I know, but we have to try." I give him a gentle squeeze on his arm—my friend.

Even though she is homeschooled, Kamy still detests school. I selected homeschool for my children before I ever conceived them. I felt that what I could offer them from home in the education arena would far surpass what they received at a public institution. I envisioned museum trips, poetry reads, zoo outings, travels to historic locations, real hands-on experiences that would help to shape them into well-rounded individuals capable of contributing to the betterment of our world. I promoted the benefits of homeschooling to Steve's and my doubtful parents and friends who believed such a lifestyle crippled my daughters' ability to grow and develop socially. I knew, however, that the life offered them through receiving such an unconventional education made them more mature. It didn't inhibit their growth as human beings, but helped them to flourish and thrive.

Before Kamy fell ill, she loved school. By the time she entered kindergarten, she read books with fervor, tackled math problems with ease, and spelled better than any other child her age. Today, the same girl does not appear in the school room. The young woman who arrives each morning now is agitated, angry, uncomfortable, and disconcerted by the prospect of facing another school day. Kamy doesn't lack intelligence, testing at or above average on all intellectual levels, but she lacks any discipline or drive. That, coupled with her arrested emotional and social development, makes educating her a daunting task.

School frustrates her every day, her concentration interrupted by the continual stream of misplaced thoughts running through her head. Kamy likens the endless stream of chaos in her head to clutter, her mind an attic crammed with artifacts decades old that still cling to some hope of existence in the light of day. They fight to stay alive amongst the introduction of new thoughts and concepts entering the space at an alarming pace. Imagine trying to navigate a convoluted maze—boxes of ancient holiday decorations, bags of old clothes, bins filled with broken toys, stacks of books long forgotten and covered in a thick layer of dust, and endless rows of memories piled high—in such a small and dark space. This is what it is like for Kamy—every day.

Her lack of awareness and ability to express herself in a constructive and appropriate manner, combined with her volcanic mood eruptions and muddled thoughts, creates an unstable blend set to explode at any given moment. When she cannot grasp a concept, she breaks her desk, slams her laptop, screams and runs down to her room where she stands on her bed and bangs on the ceiling. She slams her bedroom door, breaks it off its hinges with the force of her thrust. Kamy cannot work through a problem with composure and self-assuredness; she acts upon her first instinct—rage. Jordan weathers her storms, completing her schoolwork in the midst of the confusion. Our dogs run in fear, wary to stay clear of her wrath. At times, she kicks them in order to alleviate her anger. School remains one of her triggers, and as a result, we all stay on our toes throughout the school day, ready at any moment for Kamy to detonate.

Today, after recovering from her math meltdown, Kamy frets over writing her first research paper, a concept new to her repertoire. Her face crumples and she starts to cry. "I don't like change, Mommy. I don't understand!" I want so much to reach out and stroke her hair, gather her in my arms, comfort her, but I can't. She does not let anyone touch her—ever. I hug Jordan several times a day, giving her kisses atop her head; I do not get to indulge my devotion to Kamy in such a manner. I am emotionally segregated from my child.

I stymie my urge for affection, instead choosing to quell the escalating situation. "Kamy, everyone has to learn to perform research and write papers on their findings. The farther you progress in school, the more I expect of you." Such a statement would draw gasps from Kamy's therapists and doctors, for they decided long ago that her level of success in life is minimal at best. I recall them telling me not to worry too much about making her complete her schoolwork: "What is she going to do, Janna, go to college? A minimum wage job is realistically the most we hope for her. Even then, if she spirals into a manic phase and does not show up for work or forgets to take her medication and attacks a coworker, then what?" Most suggest placing her in special education in public school, a flawed system ill-equipped to deal with mentally and emotionally disabled children.

Special education and mental health care in Colorado is a wasteland where special-needs children are shuffled from one institution to the next as they continue to slip further away from salvation. Overworked and underpaid staff fight just to keep a lid on the tumultuous environment, unable to address the specific needs of each child. I fear placing Kamy into the public school system; it would chew her up and spit her out, unable to handle the extremes of her existence. Kamy's defiance, mood swings, propensity to violent outbursts, lack of any inhibitions, and apathy toward others seals her doom in a regimented school system, her voice lost. Am I supposed to set myself up for her failures, accepting the fact that she will never accomplish anything? I refuse.

Despite her debilitating illnesses, I expect Kamy to follow rules, live a productive life, learn, and contribute to the betterment of society at whatever pace she maintains. True, these concepts look different than others' expectations for their children, but I expect things from her all the same. Kamy contributes daily to the betterment of our family. While I struggle to cope with her illnesses on a daily basis, I cannot imagine a world without her or the remarkable contributions she makes to my life. Throughout history, individuals suffering from mental illness made dramatic impacts on the world, placing their footprints upon the mosaic of humanity. Imagine a world without the works of Virginia Woolf, Beethoven, John Keats, Tennessee Williams, or Ernest Hemingway. What would have become of our country without the leadership of Abraham Lincoln? These significant people are but a few who suffered from chronic mental illness. They exist as proof of the capability of the mentally ill. Granted, these individuals were high functioning, but the fact remains that their capabilities far exceeded the expectations of those placed upon the mentally ill. When first faced with a lifetime of caring for my daughter, I cursed God, myself, the world, anyone who would listen, for her incapacitated state. When I finally stopped blaming and started looking at my daughter, observing her world, I truly understood the magnificence of her life.

I continue to homeschool despite the hardship it creates. I refute the opinions that her life is worthless because of something beyond her control. I believe in her ability, though it may take more time to unearth her potential than it would with others, who do not suffer from developmental and mental illness. Like a delicate rose blossom, I continue to fold back the soft petals to expose the rich aroma and exquisite beauty hidden within: the incredible art she creates, her kind words when she comforts Jordan after a spill on her bicycle, the moments when she lets me touch her hand, her musical laugh when Steve tells her a joke, fleeting moments of grace. Deep within her beats a heart clear and strong, and as long as I live, I will never let her forget her significance in this world and her ability to succeed. We fight this war together. Forever I remain at her side.

My Daughter's Fate

Sleep, child, dream,
the sun is gone. The moon
slips in beside you, gaze
locked on your baby picture

tacked to the wall. It's impossible
to keep you from pain. Forgive
me. I see you naked, young
and scared. I want to run

and embrace you. I never deny
you anything, tell myself
this is not you: concrete mask, vacant
eyes, every gesture mechanic—

rigid. I need to find you
in this disguise, trapped inside
the parody. I look
in the mirror, find you housed

within me. Without knowing, I always
believed in you. You awaken the stranger
in my reflection. I promise
to love you this way, or not at all.

Today, I have a reprieve from our weekly therapy sessions. We attend therapy every week for two hours, in addition to frequent medicine checks and testing appointments. Our social lives do not exist. Adventure for our family consists of weekly excursions to the grocery store, outings to the park, or hiking with the dogs. Steve and I have not had a night to ourselves in years. Recently, Kamy's psychologist asked us, "What do you do for yourselves to recover from the exhausting task of caring for a special-needs child? Do you have any friends you lean upon?"

Steve and I burst out laughing. "We haven't had friends in years." Most of our friends and family dispersed with the wind, drifting away on sanctimonious breezes. Kamy's circle of caregivers are our closest companions.

Many people feel uncomfortable in Kamy's presence, unsure of how to respond to the multitude of her idiosyncrasies. Others feel compelled to educate us on our inadequacies as parents. Some buy into the stigma surrounding the mentally ill: child molesters, serial killers, social deviants, maniacs who climb into towers with AK-47s, picking off dozens with their keen eye and deft hand. I see people stare every day; I watch people shy away from her, wondering why a teenager requires her mother to guide her through a crowded store like a tiny child, or why she stands wailing in the aisle begging for a toy.

I recall my mother telling me after my brother shunned my family and opted for benightedness as opposed to enlightenment about Kamy's condition, "He just doesn't understand, Janna." She excuses his decision to pretend as though I don't exist. He understands all too well, as do so many others, understands the discomfort, embarrassment, and distrust most feel in the presence of the mentally ill. They do not know the truth; they cannot see past the disease.

Portrait

angry
being
hungry
girl
restless
void
ruined
woman
buried
treasure
torn
doll
heartbreaking
shame
broken
child
mad
sister
defiant
slave
deranged
mind
empty
vessel

forgotten
individual
tragic
accident
crazy
stranger
absent
spirit
destroyed
hopeless
darling
clever
visionary
genuine
living
soul
anxious
diseases
consumed
creation
fallen
angel
innocent
daughter—disappeared

Kamy's therapists and doctors encourage us to enroll her in art classes so as to emphasize her strengths. They purport art as not only an activity to soothe her, but something at which she excels as well. We call art schools, the YMCA, any community facility offering general art classes, even private sessions, in search of a place for Kamy to receive some instruction. Each organization, when told of Kamy's circumstances, politely declines to offer their services to our family. Faced with the prospect of dealing with someone who suffers from such a spectrum of mental and developmental diseases, most opt to turn tail and run in the other direction. Just as with every other idea we attempt to help Kamy expand beyond the barriers created by her diagnoses, art class fails.

Throughout the day, I try to find time to complete my work as well. I recently graduated with my bachelor's degree in English, and now work to finish my Master's of Fine Arts in Creative Writing. Truth be told, I wish I could return to simple days and a life uncluttered. When I left school almost two decades ago in order to care for my family, I never imagined myself here now at thirty-nine. Yet, life never turns out how we expect. My return to school stems from my need to provide financially for my child. A single income does not cover the years of care and treatment Kamy requires; therefore, I rise to the occasion and fulfill my responsibility.

Every day, I crouch in the corner of our small bedroom in a folding chair at a table that serves as my makeshift desk. I grind away the hours stroking my keyboard, crafting my thoughts and observations into text. I love writing; my passion for the written word runs deep, an intricate piece of my soul. Today, however, the drain of the confrontations takes a toll on my ability to think, fire rages behind my eyes with exhaustion's flames, and Kamy's at the door again, asking when she can be finished with her schoolwork for the day and play on the computer. "Mommy, when can I be done with school? It's three o'clock. Can I play now? Mommy?"

Intolerable! I have no patience left; the well runs dry. "I want you to pick up your desk before you play," referring to the mountain of papers, pencil shavings from the dozen times she sharpened the same pencil today, a bottle of lotion she carries everywhere, and a small pile of gum wrappers, evidence of Kamy's latest obsession: chewing gum. She chews several pieces of gum each day during school, convinced that it helps her think. Thank goodness for sugarless.

"My desk is picked up. I want to play!" I can hear the agitation in her voice; her anger creeps in to take part in our conversation. She sets out on a rampage I must diffuse with haste before it gets out of hand. I set aside my mountain of work, knowing that we will meet again in the dead of night.

Time for my work begins when Kamy goes to bed. From eleven at night until four thirty in the morning, every day, I write. While others sleep, I work. The night offers me asylum ever since we found a medication combination that helps Kamy sleep through the night, free from night terrors and voices in her head. I use this time of silence to create. Sometimes, however, deadlines and due dates require me to work during the day. This does not mean, however, that Kamy allows for such an indulgence of sunlight on my behalf. Today, she refuses to leave me alone. I put my computer into sleep mode on the desk. I can't bother with writing now, Kamy's waiting.

I find her hunkered down in a chair in the living room, scowling, her iPod earphones shoved in her ears. We recognized long ago the soothing aspect of her iPod. It diverts her focus to listening to her favorite songs and soothing tones as opposed to the negative reel spiraling in her mind. I wave to get her attention. "If you help me pick up your desk, you can play until dinner." I feel a bit like a pushover, but I learned long ago that you must abandon what you think is the correct way to raise a child when your daughter is mentally ill. Instead, you wing it and come up with whatever solution helps you to get through the day unscathed. She smiles and peels herself out of the chair.

"Okay!" I quell the flames again.

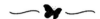

Later in the afternoon, Kamy approaches me with yet another of her relentless requests, "Mommy, can we go to the mall to get my ears pierced?" Kamy wants to pierce her ears in the worst way. She sees the fun and colorful earrings her sister wears: plump polar bears that dangle from her lobes, neon-colored happy faces, delicate gold hearts. Kamy thinks about it constantly; she spends hours devising how to make this dream a reality, but in the end, she cannot go through with the procedure.

The barriers that stand before her have nothing to do with any physical ailment or external factor that prohibits the piercing. She sleeps with blankets on her head; I told her for the first weeks after piercing, she has to leave the blankets off as they could snag on the earrings and pull them out. She can't. Kamy's mind tells her to cover her ears at night to protect them from someone stabbing her in the head. Strange? Yes. Extreme? Absolutely, but for Kamy, this is her truth. Simple changes in barometric pressure from a passing thunderstorm send her reeling; how can I expect her to handle something as disruptive to her environment as changing a part of her body?

I get so frustrated. I don't understand why she cannot overcome what I view as trivialities. When I find myself slipping into this frame of mind, I pause. I consider Kamy and the fact that her mind does not function in the same way as mine. Although her truth does not mirror mine, it is still her reality, and I ask myself, when faced with a decision over earrings or mental peace, what would I choose? I distract her, trying to put a hiccup in the loop continually streaming in her mind. "I'll think about it, okay? Why don't you go back to playing?" Her shoulders slump, and she stands with her bottom lip turned out, clutching her Captain America figure to her chest.

"Let me know soon, okay? Maybe we can go tomorrow." As she walks away, I exhale, thrilled that I avoided another confrontation, certain that I will encounter the same inquiry tomorrow, if not later that same evening.

This scenario is typical in our lives, as each day with Kamy presents a fresh challenge. Like many with mental diseases, her mind is a kaleidoscope, ever shifting in the changing light. She exists along the spectrum of instability, some days more tolerant for her than others. People challenged with mental illness and developmental disorders use coping mechanisms that can be alarming to us "neurotypicals," those who do not suffer from any form of brain irregularities.

I recall watching *Taxi* when I was little, giggling at the eccentric actions of Latka Gravas, played by comedian Andy Kaufman. His quirky behaviors provided me with endless entertainment. I didn't realize the suffering and pain taking place behind his facade. In conducting research about Kamy's illnesses, I learned that Kaufman, suspected of having Asperger's syndrome, endured a difficult childhood. He acted out his own television shows alone in the nether regions of the playground, much to the ridicule of his classmates. For them, this odd ritualistic behavior defied their concept of normalcy: playing baseball, chase, and tag like other children engaged in appropriate social interaction. For Kaufman, and so many others who fall along the autism spectrum, this action provided him comfort in a world he found over-stimulating and extreme.

Kamy engages in these same types of self-soothing behaviors that make many uncomfortable as they do not understand the purpose they serve. Kamy carries a doll or stuffed animal with her wherever she goes. Kamy picks her nails and the skin surrounding the nail bed to the point they bleed whenever she experiences any level of stress. She rubs her nose continually while she speaks. She can't go to sleep unless she repeats the same phrase to me each night, with her bedtime music that she's had since she was a baby at the exact same volume level. These rituals, the idiosyncrasies that drive me mad, serve a specific purpose: to calm the raging mind.

As the evening wears down, I prepare for the final ritual of the day. Stomach full of a chicken dinner and her evening medication, Kamy again traverses the toils of personal care. Jordan romps around in her cotton-candy-pink fleece robe awaiting her shower, our miniature dachshund nipping at her feet. Her laughter tinkles like a wind chime twisting in the breeze. I love her exuberance and wit. "I love my Mimi!" she sings, using the nickname she gave me when she was a toddler. I wish I could bottle her enthusiasm, her zeal for life; I could make a fortune. Meanwhile, Kamy wanders around looking lost, awaiting my string of commands that walk her through her process. "Kamy, go in and use the bathroom and brush your teeth so you can take a shower." Every day.

After she undresses, Kamy realizes that she forgot to bring her deodorant from her room upstairs to the bathroom. She proceeds to walk downstairs sans any clothing covering her body except her underwear. Kamy lacks any inhibitions, unconcerned with parading her naked body around our house. I must remind her every day to not walk around without clothes covering her. "You need to have some modesty. It is not appropriate for a young woman to walk around naked in front of others." She looks at me with her usual blank stare, clothed in nothing but a Yankees hat with her iPod clipped to it. *Wonderful*, I think, *she has no idea what I mean.* Just because I repeat myself constantly to Kamryn does not mean she grasps what I say. Talking to her is akin to throwing a wet towel against a wall, sometimes it sticks, but most of the time it slides off, crumpling to the ground.

I still help Kamy bathe. I am sure most find this bizarre, but for our family, it is all a part of the routine. Every small task overwhelms her, even something as mundane as blow-drying her hair, and without some assistance, she struggles to complete such tasks. Even though she uses an electric razor, Kamy still manages to cut herself shaving because she presses the razor too hard against her skin, rendering the protective cover helpless under the weight of her force.

When she started menstruating at twelve, I prepared for the worst. I knew this drastic change to her body would cause her great anxiety, and I worried about her ability to cope with this new situation, let alone care for her maturing female form. Two years later, I still find myself explaining the workings of the female body to her, as each time she starts her period, she flies into a panic, certain that something is wrong with her. I have to put sanitary pads in her underwear for her. If I don't she puts them on wrong and ends up having accidents in her pants, or worse, in her bed. I wonder how ridiculous I look standing in the bathroom with her while she sits hunched on the toilet, putting her underwear on so I can correctly place the pad inside them.

Through continued repetition, I seek to teach her the skills to help her gain some amount of independence. If I don't walk her through every step of a daily routine, she becomes lost, confused, and in turn explodes with frustration. It remains vital that I am an integral part of her life. I tell her to wash all of her nooks and crannies, and then I help wash her hair. We use a special shampoo that removes buildup from deposits left from her medication that can cause thinning of her hair. Dear God, I could never tell her that. She already thinks she's going bald. We proceed through the rest of the ritual: blow dryers, lotion bottles, and pajamas, my rites of ceremony.

Every night after showers, we say prayers before the girls watch television. Kamy then proceeds to the basement to watch her favorite shows. She carries a vast assortment of goodies that soothe her aching mind: a box of pencils, her watch, a gratitude journal that her therapist requires her to keep in which she writes the same thing every day: *I'm grateful for the nice weather. I'm grateful for watching movies. I'm grateful for getting to play on the computer.* She also carries a calculator, scissors, paper, drawing books, the hat she wore that day, a bottle of lotion, two rubber bands, a tube of hydrocortisone cream, and finally, a piece of anorexic paper, worn thin by her anxious grasp, listing all of the things not wrong with her, signed by Steve and me. We wrote the list as a matter of self-preservation. It includes topics we address with her every day, several times a day. Now, instead of having to ask us, she refers to her list:

❧ *There are no carbon monoxide issues in our home.*

❧ *It is okay for you to see circles, fog, haze, and other anomalies in your field of vision from time to time. Your eyes are not perfect.*

❧ *It is normal for you to experience headaches and discomfort around your scalp and cranium from time to time. Everyone gets headaches. Stop worrying and maybe they will go away.*

❧ *It is normal to feel your pulse or heartbeat at different locations on your body. If you feel a pulse, you are living.*

❧ *People get aches and pains throughout their body on a regular basis. You have them unless you are a machine. If you are a machine, we need to know.*

❧ *There are no gas leaks in our home. We thoroughly inspected it and are confident that no leaks exist.*

❧ *Brain tumors are extremely rare and cause side effects that you do not possess. If you are experiencing discomfort in your head, look at the previous point addressing headaches.*

❧ *Your lungs work fine.*

❧ *You are not exposed to dangerous chemicals.*

❧ *There is nothing wrong with your stomach.*

❧ *Your heart operates normally.*

❧ *It is okay to be tired. It does not mean that you are dying.*

❧ *You do not have lice.*

❧ *You are not pregnant. If you do not want a belly, exercise more.*

❧ *There is nothing wrong with your mouth or teeth.*

❧ *You are not going blind or deaf.*

❧ *You do not have cancer.*

❧ *You are not going to have an accident.*

❧ *You are not dying.*

❧ *Cross our hearts, hope to die, stick a needle in our eyes.*

Call it her survival pack; she does not go anywhere without it.

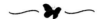

Kamy sits on the same spot on the couch every night, no exceptions, with the same blanket, pillow, and array of stuffed friends. Some wonder if allowing her to watch television before she goes to bed stimulates her already overactive mind too much, but if you walk in my shoes for one day, you see why I count the minutes until I deposit her in front of the colored screen. Besides, no amount of television viewing adversely affects her brain any more than the chemical imbalances that already mutated her gray matter. Does that make me a bad mother? In other's eyes, perhaps, but I do the best with what tools I possess.

Bedtime mercifully comes, but not before our final passage into repose. Putting Kamryn to bed is an ordeal. While the rest of us wait, Kamy begins her long and arduous preparation for bed like a surgeon preparing for the most difficult operation. She washes her hands again, and then proceeds to place every animal and blanket in their assigned location. She places exactly ten Kleenexes under her pillow and arranges her bottles of lotion, watch, and rubber bands in the same geometrical pattern on her nightstand. The volume of her bedtime music remains at the same level every night, no exceptions. If her over-stimulated hearing detects the slightest variation of tone, she demands the readjustment of the knob. I perform a final incantation to bring her into slumber:

"Goodnight Mommy."

"Goodnight Kamy."

"I love you."

"I love you too."

"Special place?"

"Go to your special place."

"Nothing is wrong with me?"

"No."

"I'm tired."

"Then go to bed." Every night, the exact same words repeated—Kamy's mantra. She rejects sleep unless I perform this last request. A final shout escapes her as I walk upstairs.

"Goodnight."

"Goodnight Kamy."

"Nothing is wrong with me?"

"No, go to bed." Every day.

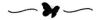

Night cloaks me in its embrace—my time. I settle down to eat my dinner at ten, more than twelve hours since I last ate. I never cook for myself. Having exhausted all of my efforts preparing the family meal hours earlier, I get takeout. I have not eaten a proper sit-down meal in years. I spend mealtime buzzing around the kitchen like a fly on crack, retrieving seconds for everyone, measuring portions, washing dishes, helping Kamy when she spills something for the hundredth time. I prefer to eat later—alone.

Dinner for me is the same every night: a footlong veggie sandwich from Subway. It's my tradition: spinach, tomatoes, pickles, banana peppers, avocado, light mayo, and salt and pepper on wheat bread. The benign flavor, the blandness, the ubiquity of my meal defies the culinary logic of most. Why not spice things up with a hummus and eggplant sandwich drizzled with basil pesto, or even better, a bowl of vegetarian chili? At least toss some jalapeños on the sandwich for a kick. How do I eat the same thing every day? The answer is simple: I crave smallness, stability, routine. My sandwich grounds me; it prevents me from flying into oblivion. In my chaotic and unstable life, sliced vegetables wedged between pillows of soft bread offer me comfort, familiarity. My life to the outside world seems plain, mind numbing, lackluster, but for those who experience a fraction of what occurs inside the barrier of these walls, a veggie sandwich every night doesn't sound too bad.

I sit and enjoy the silence, Steve next to me typing away on his computer as he catches up on his work from the day, my dogs resting at my feet. Gratitude comes in the simplest form. I am grateful for the quiet house, thankful that Kamy finds some peace now where she once lay tormented by transparent demons who whispered terrible things to her in the shadows. I am grateful for Jordan, the joy of my life. She reminds me every day of the beauty and grace found in the smallest things. I am honored to be her mother. I am thankful for Steve, who makes me laugh through my tears, who stands by my side through the misery and grief, who shares my life, for better, for worse, until death do us part. I am thankful for life, for wisdom, for strength. I glance down at my wrist, a small silver cuff bracelet surrounds it, with the word *Strength* etched upon it in English, Spanish, and Chinese. The silver is worn and scratched, some of the letters stripped of the black paint that fills the etchings, evidence of its survival. This bracelet signifies the core of my spirit, reminds me of what I need to survive this mountain placed at my feet—strength. I wear it every day.

I sit in a small metal chair next to Kamy. The fluorescent lights above us flicker in a random pattern of flashes as though to send some kind of Morse code: "Help . . . please . . . rescue . . . me." Dead flies and moths lay in a wasteland across the cover of the fixture, desiccated forms trapped in perpetual flight, their wings a silhouette against the plastic film. "Just breathe in and out," I tell her as I stare into her soft blue eyes, absent any look of understanding; she's lost.

She clutches her Selena Gomez doll in one hand and her stuffed chocolate Labrador retriever Tyrone in the other. She won't let me hold her hand, or touch her arm in comfort; anything I provide is done from a safe distance. She doesn't let me touch her, and if I do, I have to prepare her for it first, tell her that I am about to touch her and not to yell at me, just like I did when I applied the cream to her arm. "The numbing cream really works. I don't feel anything," she tells the tech again for the sixth time. "Charon prescribed it for me."

She's loud, her voice brash; an agitated tone hides just beneath the surface. I smile at the lab tech, who looks perplexed by her odd comments.

"It's Lidocaine," I tell her. "Charon is her psychiatric nurse that provides her medication. She ordered the blood draw." I am used to explaining her irregular behaviors to others who are not exposed to mental or developmental illness on a regular basis. She smiles at me with understanding and turns to Kamy.

"That's great," the young woman says as she removes another vial of garnet fluid from a shaft attached to a needle buried deep in the crook of Kamy's arm and inserts another. "Last one, okay?"

Kamy nods. "This numbing cream really works."

"Yes, Kam, it does."

We leave the laboratory, Kamy with her Selena Gomez doll in a vice grip, backpack with Tyrone the chocolate Lab hanging out strapped tight across her back. "The cream really helped. I didn't feel anything," she tells me again.

"That's great, Kamy. Get yourself hooked into your seatbelt," I instruct her as I unlock the car.

"My arm's numb," she says, frowning as she rubs her arm back and forth.

"It's okay," I assure her as I look at her from the rearview mirror, "remember, that's what it's supposed to do."

She smiles and hugs her doll to her chest. "Right."

We drive home listening to her favorite music station, the trauma of her blood draw long past, at least until the next time. I realize in this moment how grateful I am to have her in my life, not just because she is my daughter, but for what I learn from her. She helps me to dismantle my fear of what I do not understand. She reveals to me the overlooked characteristics of the mentally ill that lie buried beneath the heaps of stereotypes and misconceptions. She allows me to love her, teach her, and experience life with her. She invites me into her world. Through Kamy, I learn compassion, empathy, and grace.

I drove past a woman at a bus stop the other day; she held an empty grocery bag in her hand, pacing back and forth—yelling. No one else was with her; she argued with the air. I think back to a time where such behavior sent my sarcastic sense of humor into overdrive, before I understood the depths of mental illness. Now, I see her through new eyes, the gaze of a mother with a mentally ill child. I see someone's daughter, sister, or wife ravaged by disease. I see the loss, sadness, and denial, but beyond that, I recognize the person dwelling beneath the layers of illness, the person aching to release her voice into the world. Just like my daughter, this woman has a place in the scope of the universe's divine plan. The simple fact that she reaches her destination through altered means does not detract from the significance of her life, the impact she has upon the world, or the important role she plays in the lives of others. Outward appearances do not dictate the soul dwelling within.

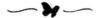

Kamy's medication causes erratic metabolic shifts. The chemicals spike her hunger while simultaneously slowing her body's response to the increased caloric intake. In my efforts to battle her weight gain, I offer up an exercise regimen that works her body. She hates any type of physical exertion; a workout for her consists of manipulating a cursor around her computer screen. With the powerful psychotropic medications she takes, coupled with the impact they may have on her long-term health, I have no choice but to force her to exercise. I also hope to stimulate some desire to take part in a "normal" activity, to strive and be like other kids her age.

Some days, I take her into the basement and send her through a half-hour aerobic routine incorporating plyometrics and calisthenics, among other high-intensity exercises, which prove most challenging for her. Asperger's inhibits a sufferer's coordination. This is the case with Kamy. I watch her contort her body in odd configurations, a pretzel gone wild. She has no rhythm and no sense of timing when it comes to performing physical feats. Jordan, who joins us in the routine, demonstrates her flexibility and skill. "Great punch kick combo, Jo," I tell her as she follows along during a kickboxing segment. I turn and see Kamy, baseball hat flopping, flailing about a bit like someone swatting at a swarm of angry wasps. Her bright red and sweaty face indicates the anxiety stirring within. I try to boost her confidence. "Keep it up, Kam!"

"I can't!" She wails and runs out of the room, slamming her bedroom door behind her.

Times like this, when she screams at me that her legs burn or her heart is going to stop or she can't do any more, I tell her in a calm voice, "Pain lets us know we're alive." I want her to know that being uncomfortable does not always equate something negative happening, a lesson that falls upon deaf ears.

Today, with the splendid weather, I decide to take everyone on a mile run. "Put on your shoes and grab your iPods. It's magnificent outside, so we're going running for our exercise today." Jordan leaps into action while Kamy drags herself from her desk chair and trounces downstairs to retrieve her shoes, displeased with my chipper announcement. We exit the house and gather on the front porch, where I give my pre-run speech. Like a coach before game time, I try to rally my troops, sending their excitement flowing while still keeping them within the parameters of acceptable behavior. "I'll run ahead of you to help you keep pace." I look at Kamy. "This is not a race. We all are doing our best. If someone passes you, we don't yell at them or get upset, okay?"

"Okay, Mommy."

"I'm going to touch you now," I announce as I reach out and straighten her fuchsia and gray Baltimore Ravens hat sitting cockeyed on her head. "Let's go!"

I take off at a steady pace; Steve and the girls follow. I continue past neighboring houses and onto a paved walking trail. I keep turning as I run to check on the others' progress. Steve chugs along at a good rate with Jordan not far behind, light on her feet like a woodland sprite. About twenty yards behind them, Kamy slogs along, her feet shuffling beneath her in an odd and disjointed cadence. She thrusts her feet to the ground with each stride, her arms stiff and robotic at her side. Kamy runs with such forced pressure and heavy foot that she eradicates the treads on brand-new tennis shoes, tearing the soles clean off. As I watch her, my heart breaks; what stranger observing this scenario would not snicker, mock her for her odd behavior and appearance? As her mother, I cannot conceive the torment that others who do not find themselves sheltered by the sanctuary of their family endure. How can they ever transcend the stereotypes, the humiliation, and the intolerance in such a hostile environment?

I read a story online recently about Donna Williams, a woman who suffered from Asperger's, and her experiences on the outskirts of society. Donna's mother slapped her repeatedly whenever Donna engaged in self-soothing behaviors, or felt she was being rude because she could not interact with other people. Donna lived for years without notice—invisible. Not even her own family understood the complexity of her mind, or the pain she suffered from her segregation from the "regular" world.

I understand Donna's mother's reaction; I empathize with her plight. Kamy's self-soothing behaviors annoy me. Her rituals make me want to run screaming down the street. And when Kamy is manic, banging her head against the wall in anger, breaking her door off its hinges, slapping her sister, screaming like a feral child, or punching her father in the stomach, I want to shake her until she stops. I want to make her feel as horrible as she makes those around her feel when she slides into her darkened state, but I pause, I take a breath, and I remember. I remember Donna's story. I remember how confusing it must be to live in a world that does not conform to your concept of reality. I remember the variances in her mind, the misfiring synapses, the chemical imbalances, and the vast chasm that exists between my truth and hers. Finally, I remember that I am her mother and she is my daughter, stripped of all of her outbursts and quirks, her diagnoses and misinterpretations, the love of my life.

On an exquisite late September Colorado afternoon—one of those days when summer still clings to late-blooming lilies glowing tangerine, lawn mowers feast on leaves dusting grass still asserting its presence and autumn steals away sunlight—I gather everyone in the car and head for the mall. For most families, an afternoon trip to the mall does not constitute a milestone achievement, but for us, any time we emerge from the safety of our inner sanctum and survive, well, it's significant. In the confines of our home, I can pretend I have a regular family, that my daughter is "normal" by societal standards. I can make believe I am in a tunnel, my blinders adjusted to block out anything that attempts to sneak into my peripheral gaze. In the light of day, I cannot ignore the truth blazoning a path of unforgiving brutality; I cannot deny the progression of my daughter's illnesses.

We wander through tiled hallways flanked on either side by various shops and boutiques. Jordan, ever the fashion diva, jostles my arm. "Mommy, can we go into Claire's?" she asks, her eyes ablaze with anticipation over perusing the endless racks of baubles and trinkets suitable for any tween.

"Sure, Bean," I smile and squeeze her shoulder. I turn to Kamy. Her hands are shoved into jeans that reach to the floor. Forced by her expanding belly, I buy her larger sized jeans that fit her waist but dip well below the natural length of her legs. Her white t-shirt stretches across her paunch; the silhouette of her belly button pressed against the fabric peers out like an orb, her flaxen hair shoved under another baseball hat. "Hey, Kam, you want to come in with us?" Shoulders slumped, she gazes across to the sports apparel store beckoning to her with its NFL jerseys and a extensive collection of hats.

"I don't like that kind of stuff. Can I go look at hats instead?"

I sigh; I'm in no mood to argue. "Sure. Steve, will you take her across to the hat store?" I watch them depart before Jordan and I walk into Claire's.

Hoards of chatty girls swallow us; they congregate around turnstiles crammed with earrings, gape at Technicolor scarves draped from the walls, giggle and swoon by the Justin Bieber merchandise. *My goodness*, I think to myself, *it's like his shrine.* I chuckle, amused with their adoration as I recall my own teenage angst, pining away over my *Tiger Beat* magazine that contained a gallery of photographs of Tom Cruise, Scott Baio, and Rob Lowe. I watch Jordan as she selects an assortment of jewelry for purchase, careful to color coordinate earrings with a charm bracelet adorned with miniature depictions of the Eiffel Tower. She glances at me and grins, the brackets from her braces shining in the fluorescent lighting. I recognize the signs of a little girl's transformation into a young woman.

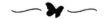

Little Girl

I pack the box
myself, pack it full
of tears: a tiny pink teddy,
It's a Girl *scrolled across belly*
plump with batten filling, a wisp
of honeyed hair soft as dandelion
fluff clipped from her head,
Hello Kitty earrings purchased
when she pierced her ears,
the first tooth she lost
on our trip to Durango. Place it
on a shelf in the back closet
beside Alice and the Mad Hatter,
late night whispers under a cloak
of blankets, and lazy morning
blueberry pancakes wet with warm
syrup; giggles season
the Sunday funnies.

Somewhere in shadows, little
girl waits for me, gold hair
woven——ribbons streaming.
We lie in grass fingers
tickling our feet like a thousand
frenzied butterflies, sculpting clouds
with our eyes: lambs, rabbit's
tails, cotton crocodiles without
legs. Rapture a kiss
on her forehead, orange blossom
clinging to velvet skin.
The house reeks
of silence. Phantom footsteps
echo in moss covered
hallways, no laughter outside
the kitchen window, tossing stones
across hopscotch games, chasing
dragonflies through flowers
thriving in glass domes. I line
drawers with letters I'll never
send: Dear sweetheart, I am a book
with no ending, a broken

guitar string, a piano absent
melody. *She is a sliver of ice*
on my tongue, last ray of sunlight
slicing the sky before dusk, pause
of a hummingbird wing. I embrace
the past when her childhood
was not yet over and time stretched
before me a flawless beach,
sands smoothed by the wave's
caress. Nothing prepared me.
When she slipped
from my branches, only then
did I realize—tomorrow.

My smile fades. I see Kamy shuffling into Claire's looking awkward and uncomfortable; anxiety pulls at the corners of her mouth. Steve trails behind with a look of exasperation on his face. My long and lovely hallucination of normalcy comes to an abrupt halt with the escape of sound from her lips. "Mooommy," the O sound stretches from her mouth, choking my splendid moment, "they didn't have anything!" Her hat, too small to contain her thick hair, now rests on the crown of her head, resembling the headwear of a long haul trucker or a farmer after a long day on the back of his Caterpillar tractor. In the rush to shop, she neglected to wipe her mouth after her snack of a soft pretzel with cheese dip. As a result, flakes of dried cheese nestle in the corner of her mouth. For a brief moment, I wonder how easy life would be without Kamy, without all the heartache and turmoil she brings. I glance behind her where I see other mothers and daughters shopping together, laughing, smiling—bonding. I have no maternal connection to this young woman standing before me. I function for her only on a primal level, but I exist for her still the same. Without my guidance and support, no matter how trying it is to be her mother, she would end up institutionalized, homeless, imprisoned—dead.

I inhale with vigor and convince my blood pressure to lower. "Kam, I'm sure we can go to another sport store and find you a hat, okay? Let's not have a meltdown." This situation has the potential to head south quickly. I recall an incident in Old Navy when she threw a temper tantrum because I wouldn't let her buy a Hello Kitty iPod docking station.

"But, what if another store doesn't have one? I want a hat!" Tears gather in her eyes, poised like acrobats waiting to take their final dive.

"We'll find you a hat, okay?"

"Can I buy a stuffed animal instead? They sell Webkinz at the store next door." A hint of optimism mixed with desperation creeps into her voice. Dear Lord, please help me. How many times a day do I have to tell her no, to stifle her obsessive urges?

"The answer is no." How I wish I could siphon away the poison that destroys her brain.

Our therapist provided me with a letter from a participant serving on a NAMI (National Alliance on Mental Illness) panel who suffered from bipolar disorder. In the letter, he spoke of how people tried to assign purpose to his illness, to "cure" him rather than focusing upon helping him understand his own needs and how to fulfill them: "When I have had a good day, and I'm tired and want to rest, you push me harder. You see this one experience as my potential to act this way constantly. You feel the need to fix me, to make me right, but you fail to recognize me for who I am, to understand that I am different from you." This letter haunts me, for it illuminates the thoughts of every mentally ill individual.

I am guilty of those charges he describes. I try to fix Kamy, to make her align with my world. I convince myself that her life would be so much easier if she functioned like everyone else. I neglect to realize that she cannot erase her mental illness any more than I can morph into a man. It is a part of her, embedded in her DNA. Jim Sinclair, an autism activist, speaks to the concept of "modifying" the mentally ill by attempting to normalize them behaviorally: "Expecting that we learn to 'act normal' is sort of like expecting blind people to learn to drive cars instead of teaching them skills to use public transportation." Rather than trying to alter my child and extinguish her behavior deemed inappropriate, I need to accept her, understand her, and help her to exist, as she remains in a world hostile to her authenticity.

In the magical realm of the mind, anything is possible. We learn, explore, create, dream, believe, forming our existence based upon our ability to adapt our thoughts and ideas to the external world. For Kamy, and others who suffer her fate, the mind is an amusement park fun house where around every corner lurks a hidden danger: a mirror that warps reality, a dead end, an endless maze. Life is uncertain, a rocky cliff giving way under their weight. What makes their existence even more frightening is the hostilities they face in a world lacking the awareness of their variations. Kamy, like so many other mentally ill individuals, still functions on the same primal levels as any human being; they want for love, companionship, success, peace, and self-fulfillment. However, for the mentally ill, achieving these goals feels insurmountable as they wade through the chemically imbalanced clutter accumulated in their minds.

Who decides what is the forest and what is the trees, which way is up and which way is down? How do we know that our way is the "right" way? When I enter Kamy's world, I do so without any preconceived notions of normalcy. I imagine myself an outsider looking in, much as she must feel in my domain. I picture a world upside down and inside out, trapped in a Dr. Seuss book or Alice's nightmare. I immerse myself in a place both familiar and strange. I need to feel connected to her so I can provide her the environment she needs to grow and thrive to the best of her ability.

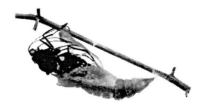

III.

Of all the rights of women, the greatest is to be a mother.

—Lin Yutang

Motherhood is not what I imagined. Of course, my vision was skewed by what I found in television shows and magazines. I wanted desperately to be the mother whom everyone admired, the one with the perfect home and the perfect children. I channeled Martha Stewart and Claire Cosby, an amalgam of strength, devotion, and exceptional domestic skills. When I found out I was pregnant with Kamy, I busied myself with every activity known to new mothers in preparation for my little miracle. I painted her room with a huge mural of Noah's Ark; bears, kangaroos, hippos, and elephants gazed out from the wall to witness her arrival. I bought tiny buckle shoes and ruffled sleepers, delicate bows fashioned with Velcro backings to secure in her downy hair. I documented every morsel I placed in my mouth, assuring I ingested the exact amounts of all nutrients and vitamins vital to a fetus's development. I read to her, sang to her, took walks every morning, plodding down the street with my dogs in tow, belly swollen, all to assure her health and prosperity. I was the vision of the perfect mother, just as I wanted.

God is humorous. He watched while I plodded about in my maternal stupor, amused by my pursuit of Utopia, unaware of what lay coiled along my path. I assumed if my child emerged from my womb with ten fingers and toes, intact in every physical aspect, then nothing else could go wrong. When Kamy arrived on a brisk November afternoon after only a four-hour labor, angels gasped, nurses swooned, and I marveled at my ability to create a flawless child. With dark blue eyes and a shock of curls haloing her exact round head, I felt like the luckiest woman in the world. I refused any medication during labor, not wanting to cause any unforeseen damage to my baby.

As I held her close to me, her lips pursed with a tiny frown as she dreamt of some unknown threat in her new surroundings, I thanked God for my little girl, everything I hoped for and imagined, unaware of what lurked beneath the small pink cap placed with care atop her head. God took my perfect family and tossed it into a hurricane, just to see where we landed. Like game pieces from a Monopoly game gone awry, he maneuvered our lives in such a way that we never could pass Go, rounding the board in an endless parade of despair and confusion. He tossed the die, leaving my daughter's life to the whim of chance.

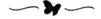

Room 402

Time is apathetic
to my misery. It crawls
along the wall, searches
for a decent program
to watch at four in the morning.
My belly blisters
and groans. Her soft fingers
brush my womb like a feather
strikes the wall. I say Amen
to her introduction, thankful
for the kind gesture. I hate
the wallpaper, lady finger pink
and little boy blue.

How do I escape fire
running wind sprints
across my stern? I thirst
for water; they bring me ice;
frozen glass tears my nerves.
Pack my night gowns,
burp cloths, and my good mother
books. I know their refrain.
I pray she doesn't turn
blue. Can she roll over
at four months, sing "Mary
Had a Little Lamb" when she
turns two?

I never asked
her name. We are strangers,
though I trace the pattern
of her elbow, knee, her plush
head. We shake hands
across a plane paper
thin. Does she hear
my voice? Tell her
I love her; She might not
know. I confuse her
when I weep dehydrated tears,
or yell to quiet her fears.
Can I unlock her
cipher? I need a cryptologist.

Stop by later
in the month,
or year, or never.
Keep her longer.
I'm not ready
to obey physics. I defy
gravity. Is she ripe?
Is she ready? She clings
to my branch too long.
I am brutal to leave her
inside. She sleeps safe
in my house, Rock-a-Bye,
don't let the bough
break. Do I spread my wings
and let her fall? Sever the string
that tethers her to me.

Please come soon,
or not if you choose.
I wait in room 402.

All That Remains

I read the books, painted the nursery
a flamingo convent with gingham
trim, played Chopin, Mozart—Mary
Had a Little Lamb. I stuffed drawers
with socks, bibs, and pacifiers
in my infinite nesting; I filled the emptiness—
waiting. I sang lullabies to phantoms, restored
the antique crib for this tiny stranger, crowned
it with a butterfly halo dancing. I choked
on peanut butter sandwiches with tomato juice
chasers, cuddled pixie shoes, lumbered through
doorways like a slow ox, my breasts
weeping. I fashioned her from love
and bone: her delicate wrists, spindle
fingers, filament lashes, soft hair
in my waters rising. I ache

for her arrival. She presses
my womb. Nothing prepares us
for the storm coming. She overwhelms
me. From the belly
of the house, I hear her
crying. Phones ringing, dogs
barking—I cannot stand
the clamor. Is it morning,
night? I lie alone, wishing
she were a fern, a flower. I can't
find her bear, bottle,
the damn ribbon to tie
in her hair. Shhh shhh, baby,
hushabye, curl up
and drift away. I toss
pennies into a barren
fountain hoping
for a tree house
scraping heaven.
Nothing remains, my
daughter.

In Case of Motherhood: Pull Cord

Motherhood: desire
to shed responsibility
like a second skin.

She bloomed from me.
I waited, crescendo of joy
building. Out came a bundle
of flesh and cord; a small
viscous lump bore all my hopes
and desires, an epiphany
swaddled in a tiny pink bundle.
Trapped inside my Ziploc
chamber, I worry the baby
will eat rat poison, drown
in the dog's water dish.
I unclog disposals jammed
with bread crust, Captain America
and onion skin, dredge the bottom
of a glass of milk and Oreo sludge
in search of the misplaced bud ready
for the Tooth Fairy.

She threw up
cherry Jello on the bedspread,
pulled a Pollack
with permanent markers
on the dining room wall.
My child soaks sheets
with the reconstituted last glass
of water before bed,
beckons me at 2 AM
to satiate her obsessions.
Like a cockroach
she overruns everything.
I am demoted from bed
to sofa, mashed potatoes crusted
in my hair. Some species
eat their young.

I read board books
about animal escapades and red
balloon sagas. Soda box pyramids

balanced on the cart tumble
in the parking lot; I forgot
where I put my keys. Plastic
stretched around milk jugs as thin
as my patience.
Wakeful
hungry
restless
screaming
crazy
I fear nothing.

Women glide by in stilettos
and Donna Karan, sparkling grace
and beauty. They sleep in silence
on silk pillows. No voice
calls for them to ward off
closet monsters. They copulate
in uptown living rooms on priceless
Oriental carpets. Who surrounds
their table at Thanksgiving,
tattoos the refrigerator
with crayon renderings?

Little fingers expand beyond
outlines scratched onto paper,
mark another notch on the wall.
What becomes of me
when this day ends?
No amount of her love
is ever enough.

I awaken each morning prepared for battle, but my spirit on this morning wavers. I am not ready to face the constant barrage of temper tantrums, outbursts, and crying marathons. When the alarm goes off, I moan; a knot tightens around my gut. My digestive system suffers a most horrid existence as it absorbs the brunt of my stress. I am agitated before I ever lay eyes on Kamy. The previous night, she exploded at bedtime because Jordan came upstairs to say goodnight to us before Kamy was ready, disrupting her ritualistic pattern. We all endured her rage for twenty minutes before she calmed herself enough to go to bed.

At breakfast, I can tell by her sullen stare and subdued demeanor that today is not going to fare well. "Daddy, don't touch me!" she yells as Steve inadvertently brushes her shoulder at the table.

"You need to calm down," I tell her in an even voice, trying to maintain my composure. "Go get dressed and ready for school." Kamy slams her chair back from the table and storms down to her room. She never yells at me, although I am her disciplinarian. She rants and spews hate in both Steve's and Jordan's directions, but never mine. It is unsettling; I know she must have pent up rage geared in my direction, but she never lets it show. I ponder waking up one night and finding her standing over my bed with a pillow.

Without missing a beat, Kamy starts her school day causing problems. Again, she complains about her work and lack of understanding. "Mommy, I don't know how to do this activity," she whines in a voice I can't stand. On this morning, it pierces my ears like someone blasting squelch from an AM radio. I pick up her notebook and glance at the blank pages, not a pencil mark in sight.

"You haven't even tried." My blood pressure reaches dangerous limits. I take a deep breath, trying to calm myself.

"They want me to find articles about freedom, but I can't find any. I don't know what I am supposed to do." Her face pinches with anxiety, the same look she gets each time right before she explodes. I am like a seismograph; I detect her eruptions with deft skill and accuracy.

"Kamy, all I ask is that you try on your own first before you ask for help. I don't ask for perfection. I just expect you to try."

"Mommy, I can't!" she squeals. "Can I have my toys sit with me? They help me concentrate." I follow her eyes to the closet; through the sliver of space between the door and the frame, I see Captain America, Selena Gomez, and various stuffed animals peering out from the crack. I quiver with rage and resentment. No longer able to control myself, I burst.

"I expect you to follow my rules. No toys during school!" I cannot remember my mantra: *Kamy is mentally ill. She can't help who she is. Forgive her flaws; walk in her shoes.* When I look at her, I see my devastation. I see a burden that consumes the air I breathe. She suffocates me, robs me of any semblance of a normal existence. I'm sick of the rituals, the tirades, the doctor appointments and therapy sessions, the time she steals that I could be spending with Jordan, the stares, my marriage hanging on by a thread, the intolerable isolation. In this moment, I hate my daughter.

Kamy's screaming and crying, hysterical over my outburst. I grab a stack of folders off the desk and swat the top of her New York Giants hat with a resounding *THWAP*. "Shut up!" I scream, unable to control my temper. "I've had enough!"

Steve comes running into the room. "What the hell is going on?"

"Daddy, help me!"

"I want her out of my house. I am sick of this. I can't take it anymore!"

Steve grabs Kamy by the arm and steers her out of the room. "Go to your room."

"I'm going to call the police on you!" she screams at him as she retreats to her room. She slams the door so hard the doorknob falls to the floor—again. I try to recover from my explosion by taking several deep inhalations, envisioning myself anywhere but trapped in this life. Purged of all my negative emotions, I feel better, for a moment, until I see Jordan looking at me from the kitchen table, where she is building a clay model of a rhinoceros.

"Look, Mommy," she says in her sweet voice, "I made this for my social studies assignment. I sculpted a piece of cave art, just like the cave people. Do you like it?" I walk over to her and admire the small blue lump with bulging eyes and misshapen legs.

I hug her to me. "I love it, Jo, you did a great job." In indulging my selfish behavior, I neglected to remember this innocent bystander. I am ashamed. God reminds me of my many imperfections. I am not an ideal mother; I'm human—flawed.

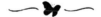

After time spent in her room, Kamy emerges refreshed, forgetting earlier events as a result of her selective memory. For her, life continues, but for me, I cannot escape the images of myself towering over her, spewing my hatred like a poisoned geyser. I slink about, riddled with guilt over my behavior. As I prepare dinner that night, Kamy comes into the kitchen. Captain America dangles at her side. "Mommy, what can I do? Jordan doesn't want to play with me."

"Kam, you don't always have to have someone play with you. Make up something on your own." I continue to peel potatoes, hoping my remarks send her back to where she came.

"I don't know how to play by myself. My brain doesn't work that way. I need someone to help me." What child doesn't know how to play? A small tear slips from the corner of my eye. My daughter, the one I curse, the one who fills me with resentment and pain, this young woman forever imprisoned in her stunted development, tortured by her twisted mind, reminds me of my humility. My ego took control of me earlier in the day. I neglected her; I forsook my responsibility to her as her mother, through all of life's pain and struggles. She does not choose to be this way—who would? She needs me, just as much as I need her. Please, God, forgive me.

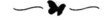

My Last Testament

What shall I leave my heiress,
a cloth blanket to cover
her indiscretions? I worry
what becomes of her.

Can you see a soul die,
leave the body in steam
rising? I feel useless
as a broken lock.

Neural pathways twist
and wind like a bowl of spaghetti.
Black wool hangs in her gray
matter, cocoons I wish wouldn't hatch.

She hides voices beneath
the pillow, paralyzed by questions
tumbling over and over like a river
polishing stones in her mind.

Tell me to pray. I beg
for a response. I wanted children
with appendages intact. I neglected
to consider the brain—the boss.

I should love her,
I'm her mother. I don't
today. I scream for years,
a simple life my only desire.

She is a miracle: two negative
numbers multiplied, double
rainbow, white bison,
my enigma. I'll never
leave her side.

My girl, I follow you
until seas run dry. When I die,
examine my heart, stone still
where you reside.

I carry my love
for you beyond time.

People often remark with amazement at how I manage to survive, even excel, at the life I lead. The answer is simple: I do it with determination, devotion, and faith; determination not to let my daughter slip into the oblivion of a failed and broken mental health system, devotion to my family and their prosperity, and faith in God and myself. In the darkness of night, Steve next to me snoring softy, I marvel at the evolution of my life. Once a woman meek and compliant, my voice a whisper of a dragonfly wing floating on the breeze, I shout, I defy, I proclaim my name—I must; I have no other choice.

We recently learned of the existence of a wait-list that determines when people who suffer from developmental disabilities receive state-funded Medicaid benefits and services. Each state has a separate list, some more apt than others at providing much-needed services to the disabled. Colorado does not fare as well as others. Kamy could remain on the list for upwards of fifteen years before she becomes eligible to receive help with life skills, housing, and employment, among the myriad of other demands she needs fulfilled. With a Social Security income maximum of seven hundred dollars, and few or no services available, the bulk of her care rests upon Steve's and my shoulders.

Sometimes, I envision myself shuffling down grocery aisles when I'm seventy, my forty-four-year-old daughter trailing behind me, clutching her Captain America doll, a backpack bursting with stuffed animals strapped to her back. I see myself cutting her hair with arthritic hands as she refuses to get her hair cut by anyone else, born from her delusional fear of someone shaving off her hair. I witness myself hunched over her bed in my basement, making sure her blankets fall just right so as to alleviate her fear of bugs scurrying from the floor into her bed, I picture driving her to her appointments because she can't drive herself (one manic episode during rush hour could prove fatal). These scenarios, though extreme and far-fetched to others, are based in the reality of a parent living with a mentally ill child.

Kamy's getting worse. Each day I feel her slip a bit further from my grasp. Like a tide rolling in, her illnesses sweep her away into dark whirlpools and endless eddies that refuse to relinquish their control over her mind. I try to reach through the fog and haze of confused thoughts and misguided emotions to that little girl with blond ringlets and serene smile I knew so long ago, but she retreats into hidden corners, pursued by the shadow men that haunt her, where I can't reach. All I can do is think about those last days before she said goodbye.

Birthday Party

Memorize her face.
We laugh, fill our bellies
with butter and strawberry jelly finger
sandwiches, lady bug tea cakes
and butterfly cookies.
Sing songs to the birthday girl
in her Dora the Explorer party hat
and patent leather shoes, blue blanket
flung around her shoulders—

Supergirl.

Explode, little bullet, jump up
and down, float high
and higher, a balloon let go.
Sunlight scatters glitter
in her hair, giggle
tinkles and twists in the wind
like a silver spoon chime.
Everyone watches, drunk
on her delight. Bounce higher,
little sprite.

Like dandelion tuft, drift
up, hands flung wide,
spin away from my failure.
My daughter—gone
forever. I did little for her.
They tell me forget
the past; I embrace it.
It keeps me whole.

The first time I tried to socialize Kamy was when she was two. I signed her up for a Tumbling Tot gymnastics class at a local venue not far from our house. I figured it was the perfect opportunity to meet some other mothers with children Kamy's age. Life as the wife of a deputy isolated me. Kamy and I both needed some human interaction. I bought her a tiny royal blue velour leotard that complimented the shade of her eyes. I told her about the planned activities weeks before her first class, trying to bolster her enthusiasm. "Kamy, when you go to class, you get to roll around on mats and jump on giant trampolines. Doesn't that sound fun?"

She clasped her tiny hands together in delight. "Yeah, Mommy!" Kamy had never been outgoing. In the presence of other children (cousins' birthday parties or work-related gatherings for Steve) she usually chose a quiet corner to play by herself. I knew this class would swing the door open wide, expose her as the bright, enigmatic child I saw.

The day of her first class, I helped her shimmy into a pair of black tights and her new leotard. "Soft," she said as she ran her small hand across the fabric stretched across her lithe chest.

"Yes, soft and fuzzy, like a teddy bear," I told her as I clipped small turquoise butterfly barrettes into the wisps of blond hair scattered about her head. "We're going to have fun!" I told her, standing back to admire my little girl.

"Yeah! Fun!"

The moment I attempted to remove Kamy from her car seat in the parking lot of the gymnasium, she started screaming, a shrill scream that shattered the atmosphere. I managed to extract her from the car and carry her inside, where the screams and wails continued. Families gathered to watch their little ones jump and roll about stood with mouths agape at the sight of this cherub equipped with the lungs of the devil. "Kamy, let's go join the others in your group," I told her. She clung to me, refusing to acquiesce to my request. I stroked her hair in an attempt to soothe her, but she pushed my hand away and continued her cries. She was inconsolable, unable to calm down in the face of having to interact with others. I knew my efforts were futile. I turned and made my way back out to the parking lot, wading through the throngs of parents and their children gathered in the entryway. I parted them like the Red Sea, each person stepping aside with haste to avoid my daughter's shrieks and spasms. I raced to our car and dropped her into her safety seat again, the same one I peeled her from only minutes earlier.

Sensing safety and isolation once more, the tirade ceased, replaced by small hiccups of air and a quivering lip. I collapsed in the driver's seat, exhausted from Kamy's escapade. I looked at her in the rearview mirror, amazed by the display put forth from such a tiny person. She sat curled beneath her favorite afghan my mother made for her when she was born, thumb jammed in her mouth, sucking with fervor. "Let's go home, okay? We'll stop at McDonald's on our way. You can get a Happy Meal."

A grin broke through her pain. She removed her thumb from her mouth and clapped. "Yeah! Fun!"

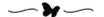

What began as the terrible twos now stretches beyond the borders of normalcy, no end in sight. This evolution into shadows hums along with precision and urgency. Her therapy sessions do nothing to make a dent in her obsessive compulsive behaviors, anxieties, or mood swings. Our family therapist could not breech her barriers after three years of trying every method she knew, so we retreated, licking our wounds as we devised a new plan. Steve and I decided to start a course of treatment with the psychologist who diagnosed Kamy, Dr. Thede. Upon our first meeting with her since she tested Kamy two years prior, she asked us to update her on the situation.

I released a torrential flood of information, recapping each horrid emotion, behavior, and mood exhibited by Kamy. At the end of my purging, Dr. Thede sat back in her chair, eyes sweeping over our faces. "So," she pondered, "it sounds as though you have your hands full. What I would like to know is what are you doing for yourselves during all of this? Taking care of a special-needs child is taxing; it takes a toll." Steve and I sat in silence, unable to fashion a response. Caring for Kamy is our life; we know of nothing else. Understanding our lack of answer to her question, she smiled. "Don't worry, we'll get through this."

Dr. Thede outlined her proposed course of treatment for Kamy and the rest of our family, an intensive schedule of therapy for us and Jordan and social and living skills development for Kamy. "Kamy has no idea how to play, to interact with others. She lacks any insight. I need to come down to her level, reach her where she is and start building from there."

How absurd, I thought, *a fourteen-year-old who has no clue how to play*. Again, I felt my old friend guilt coming to say hello. What kind of mother am I if I can't even help her share in a moment of joy with another? Kamy has no friends; how can you socialize when you have no concept of yourself, let alone others? I failed my little girl.

With each new therapy proposed, each new drug administered, each new technique implemented, my hope fades more. Each time I sit in a therapy session with a new doctor or therapist, I feel like a trained circus monkey as they send us through the same regimens as their predecessors, each one thinking their techniques will somehow cure what ails my daughter. I jump and dance for them in a grand display, doing just as they say, to no avail; Kamy remains stagnant, unchanged—the same.

Recently, we returned to our old therapist in search of some stability. Granted, Ellie, who is a family and marriage therapist, is not schooled in the nuances of dealing with an individual who contains within her a Molotov cocktail of mental deficiencies, but her empathy and understanding far outweigh our need for yet another clinician fumbling over words to try and explain the enigma of our daughter's mind. Families with chronically mentally and developmentally ill children do not need a restructuring of the same diagnosis each time they enter a therapist's or psychiatrist's office; they need a shoulder on which to lean, a comfortable place to be honest and open about the travesty that is their lives. I appreciate Ellie because she laughs with us through the pain. She doesn't judge, but rather listens with a kind heart and a keen awareness of the adversity we face, not only from Kamy's illnesses but the outside world as well as it continually heaps stigma upon our family. She sees Kamy, and the rest of us, in our authentic form: lovingly flawed.

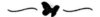

We approach the end of the path with regard to treating Kamy from home. Assisted living, or worse, hospitalization, looms not far behind me. I feel it, taste it in the acrid air. One day, soon, it will barge in, push against the door I barricade myself against with all my might. Once it infiltrates my home, nothing remains. It attaches itself to everything like the stench of stale smoke clings to fabric. Steve already buys into the lies it weaves, the deception that it offers us the answer to our problem. He tells me, "The rest of our family goes on living, Janna, even if she doesn't. If things don't improve soon, something is going to have to change." The threat hangs in the air. I imagine a cartoon bubble filled with the harsh words suspended above Steve's head, etched into the paper for eternity. I can't deny it; I know the truth—it's coming.

Recent visits to the psychologist confirm our suspicions; Kamy is trapped in a perpetual regressive state. In order to reach through the muddled confusion residing in her mind, I resort to teaching tactics I implemented with her when she was little. During our last visit, Steve and I spent the hour jotting down techniques in a notebook in an effort to try to right our floundering child. "You need to make everything concrete for Kamy. She cannot handle critical thinking, either in school or her personal life. Perhaps allowing her to draw her assignments instead of writing them will help improve her understanding," Dr. Thede told us as we sat across from her.

I felt the familiar pressure of a migraine creeping in behind my sockets. I recalled Kamy at five, first learning to read and write. I sat next to her every day while she traced letters with pencils fat and round, read about talking bears and clever pigs with timed precision, and counted numbers on her miniature fingers and thumbs. Now, almost a decade later, I faced the same existence. "I know I'm asking a lot of you, but this is what Kamy needs. You must break every skill down into a basic step-by-step process with constant repetition, every day, no exceptions."

I looked at her. She sat in her wingback chair, her laptop perched atop her legs outstretched to recline on the ottoman in front of her. She appeared so relaxed, at ease, not at all like Steve or me. I glanced at Steve; his dazed expression alerted me to the fact that he reached his maximum capacity for information regarding Kamy's extensive care.

What the hell? I thought to myself. *How do some get to lead such regular lives while the rest of us struggle?* I tried to swallow, but my mouth remained arid; my tongue clung to the roof of my mouth in an attempt to extract any moisture. *I might as well ask the million dollar question since we're on such a role,* I thought.

"Kamy will be an adult soon, and it feels as though she is getting worse, not better. Realistically, what can we expect for her?" I asked, afraid of the answer I knew lurked just beyond her lips.

"Do you mean will she ever lead an independent life?" she asked me.

"Yes."

"The answer is, we don't know. Every person along the autism spectrum is different. With Kamy's compounding issues, like bipolar disorder, certainly she faces a far more difficult road than others who have just Asperger's. If we try all of these measures, and she still is unable to grow and develop, then we can explore your other options: group homes, home care aides, there are even people who will come wake her up in the morning and get her going."

Convenient, I could use that now, I thought, bemused by her spry response laced with impending doom.

"Let's tackle one issue at a time, okay?" Right, because I have nothing but time, time to plan for my daughter's dwindling future.

Leaving our appointment that day, I found myself riddled with guilt and overwhelmed by the prospect of such intense and long-term care. I considered myself a horrible mother for neglecting my special-needs daughter, placing my desires before hers. In my effort to finish my degree so as to financially provide for her, I forgot the everyday necessities, the basic functions that I expected her to manage. Did I forget her illnesses, or did I still deny them? Perhaps I thought if I ignored them long enough, they would go away, grow their twisted spindles in someone else's psyche, not my daughter's. I grappled with reconciling the two sides of my being: the one searching for a life of her own, independent of her family, and the one forever bound to her child. Exiting the building, I noticed a sign placard on the wall next to a darkened office space: National Prayer Task Force. I peered in the window; an abandoned front desk stood sentinel over the shadows of chairs and end tables stacked with magazines. An anemic Jesus clung to a cross suspended above the work station. Not a soul stirred. *That figures,* I thought, *when I could use a hand, God takes the day off.*

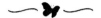

Kamy's brain is far more powerful than I ever conceived. It whispers to her, promises her things I cannot. I am defenseless in its attack on my daughter's sanity. Try as I might, I am losing the battle. Her illnesses, like the endless sky, spread across everything. Will I go into her room one day and not be able to rouse her from her bed? Will she throw her arms up in defeat, surrender to the pitch itching to consume her? What do I do with her clothes, her dolls, her hats, her blankets and toys if we have to place her somewhere? How will she make it without them? Will her caregivers know she likes ranch dressing with everything? Will they indulge her Avengers fetish with drawing tablets used to recreate her heroes? Will they ridicule her when she props her stuffed wolf against the glass door to watch while she takes a shower? Who will help her understand algebra and civics? Who will explain what it means to be compassionate, to care for others? Will they mock her odd behavior? What will they say to her each night she rambles off her nonsensical bedtime montage? Who will listen to her when she cries, when she wonders why demons plague her? Who will care? Who will come?

December 15, 2012, looms large in my mind. We were in the process of moving to a new house and Steve and I were caravanning across town in separate cars to our new location, Kamy and Jordan safely kept for the day at my mother's house.

The warmth of the December sun reflecting off the driver's side window lulled me into a stupor, dreaming of our new home and the possibility that such a move could rejuvenate our beleaguered family. My cell phone ringing jostled me from my daydreams. "Hello?"

"Did you hear about the shootings in Connecticut?" Steve asked from the other end.

"No! What happened?"

"Someone went into an elementary school and killed a bunch of kids. Turn on the radio and you can listen to the report." I hung up and switched on a local talk radio station. I spent the next twenty minutes of my drive absorbing the horror that poured from the speakers: first graders, assault rifle, showered bullets, twenty-seven dead including the gunman and his mother, history of mental illness, Asperger's—tragedy.

I wept. I cried for the lost innocence, for the children killed before they even lost their first tooth, for the brave teachers and administrators that sacrificed themselves for others, for the other teachers that locked away their students in closets and bathrooms, quelling their tiny fears with stories and games, for the first responders who witnessed the carnage, for the tiny voices screaming, "I just want to have Christmas! I don't want to die!" Selfishly, however, the one for whom I wept the most was Kamy. I feared for my daughter. How would the world perceive her now, a monster just like the killer?

Incidents like this perpetuate the stereotypes of the mentally ill: freaks, killers, molesters, abominations not fit to live among the rest of society. This is not my daughter; she is not dangerous, at least not right now. Before we found the right combination of medication she was. I know it is a reality that we can face a similar scenario again as she matures and her chemistry changes. It's possible that she, too, could snap given the right volatile mixture of brain chemistry and outside stimuli. I realize the instability of her fractured mind. Whenever Kamy hears of an incident involving an altercation, she always tells me, "I would just hit them and tell them to shut up," or "I would punch them if someone tried to tell me what to do." She makes such statements with joviality, unaware of the social, legal, and ethical ramifications of such acts. In her mind, there are no real consequences for her negative behaviors. She believes herself immune from any form of retribution, much like others who suffer her same afflictions, much like the Newtown shooter. I wonder if his mother considered if this would ever happen to her son? Why did she teach him to shoot weapons, supply him with guns if she felt he was a danger to himself and others? This is the life of the parent of a mentally ill child. We long for normalcy, so much so that we live in denial at times.

I don't know how I would handle it if Kamy ever hurt another and there was something I could do to prevent it. I hope to keep her free from the horrors of institutionalization, allow her a free and independent life, but what if she changes, grows dark and dangerous? What choice will we then have? We live in a reactive society with regard to the mentally ill, acting only in the event that they either injure themselves or others. Such a flawed system fails both the ill and the remainder of society on monumental levels. What could we prevent if we brought mental illness from the shadows into the light of understanding? I want to protect Kamy from the gawks, the stares, the insinuations, the misguided judgments, but when something like this incident occurs, how can I? What went through his diseased mind as he fired his weapon into all of those little babies, those teachers, his mother? Did he even recognize them or himself, or had the demons taken total control of him? How do I advocate for a group of people so vilified by society? How do you champion for the forgotten?

I do not mean to detract from the devastating loss, but my heart breaks as well; it breaks for my daughter and the insurmountable mountain looming before her, the summit of a normal existence free from persecution. She is not like these individuals, yet her diagnoses forever link her to them. She has no choice, and I have no choice but to be her mother. I would never turn my back on her, no matter how difficult it is to care for a special-needs child. This is not what I envisioned motherhood to be, yet here it is all the same. I know other families abandon hope, turn to a fractured system to care for their child, emancipated from the burden. I don't think I could live with myself; the guilt would consume me. Every time I get angry with Kamy or resent her presence, guilt reminds me of my duty as a mother. What kind of mother am I to blame my ill daughter for her conditions and how they impact my life? I struggle with my conscience; what would life be like free of her presence, free of the burden she symbolizes? How dare I think such vicious thoughts? At least I have my child with me, both of my daughters, safe from harm. They get to awaken each morning to a new day and will never have to experience the terror and fear that those children in Newtown did, God willing. How dare I. . . .

Broken Daughter

Keep my thoughts in order.
My mind played tricks, concealed
warning signs. I am proud
of my pain. Whisper a prayer
of my own concoction:
ill planned, muddled, carelessly
composed, an introspection
of insincerity. I don't know
what I am doing.

I'm putty in God's hands,
full of strength, etched
in fragility, broken daughter
of Eve, the flightless butterfly.
I am glad to be alone.
Close my ears to her suffered
cries; our secrets cloud the water.
One lost soul is a tragedy,
a hundred thousand is a statistic.
How lucky I am I loved her
for even a moment
before she faded.

Come in from the outside,
the two of us against the world.

Every morning, before I wake Kamy from her slumber, I pause to watch her rest. Long lashes rest upon her cheek undisturbed by anxiety, anger, or frustration. The room echoes with an unfamiliar stillness like the gathering of thunderheads before the tornado emerges. I dig into the recesses of my memory and recall rocking her in the wicker chair my father refinished for me before her birth. I see our reflection, mother and daughter, in the snow stretching into forever outside her window, a mirror in the sky. I stroke her hair; each wisp embraces my fingers. Her scent clings to my skin: apples, baby powder, and lavender shampoo. Nothing can take her from me.

I place my lips to her miniature fist and sing: *Rock-a-bye baby, on the treetop, when the wind blows the cradle will rock, when the bough breaks the cradle will fall, and down will come baby, cradle and all.* You fell, baby, far and long, but I am here to catch you. Breathe out so I may pull you in. *Thank you, God, for Kamy. Help me steady her when she falls weak, love her despite her flaws, comfort her in times of need. If she is meek, then make me strong. If she fears, grant me courage. If she weeps, let me dry her tears. If she falls silent, let me scream.*

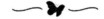

For Kamryn

I

Sleep my child, soon night
arrives. Swallow magic beans
that grow spindles of reason
in your mind.What happens,
my sweet, when the magic ends?
I dread the dark coming. I watch you
breathe, chest expands and constricts
like a snake swallowing a mouse
into its belly, and wonder
when I stopped believing
in Heaven. I hold your pieces
in my hand, puzzling, pondering
genealogy, mismatched chromosomes,
white and blue striped socks thrown
together, that created you. Some days
I wish you weren't mine, days when I blame
God for His wondrous blessing.

II

I sit bedside,
stroke your hair wet with panic
and perspiration. Dream turquoise
hummingbirds small as a bumble bee,
ride them across the buttered
sky. I wish to set myself on fire,
absorb your pain, make the voices stop
screaming. I long to rest my cheek
upon your shoulder, touch your skin
ivory and smooth as a polished
wishing stone skipped across the water.
Your flesh recoils from my touch, a rattler
set to strike; motherhood is a charade.
An army of plush animals unify
at the bottom of your bed, stave demons
creeping along the walls; glass eyes
keep watch over you as you rest.

III

I waved goodbye to the little girl
in my dreams, flaxen hair a flowing

golden eddy, eyes the blue of robin's
eggs bright and glistening, waved
so many times until nothing
remained. I remember days we watched
a color wheel rotate across the summer sky,
your hair wet and salty, seated
in our lawn chair thrones, wrapped
in your favorite Winnie the Pooh towel,
baking cookies, dough spackling
cheeks stained with curiosity, tiny fingers
searching for chocolate treasures.
My mad girl, you fear everything
but yourself: vipers entwined
beneath the covers, piranhas in bath water—
my embrace.

IV

You forget your name, soar
in and out of lucidity a wingless dove
adrift on a fickle breeze. Eyes open
and shut, detached from reality;
float in yourself, unaware.
You act strange, a little off, unscrewed,
dented—broken. Throw toys
against your splintered door, feet stomp
so loud the floors shudder.
I tell you to whisper; you scream.
I wash your hair every day, fingers stained
with my contempt. Gather your hair in bundles,
silk tendrils in my hand, scrub each tuft
with all my might; I can't scrape
the sickness away,
no matter how I try.

V

When God kicked
the chair out from under me
I cried for your ruined life, ash sifting
through my fingers. Family and friends
offer forced condolences,
purchase cards, advice
and personal tragedies strung

together like a noose
of black pearls. My house bursts
with hollow blessings. No one
can return my daughter.
They say there is nothing worse
than death; death is final. I stoop
low, enter caverns of grief,
watch you die every day.
Other mothers gather
at the wailing wall, shrouded
in pain, weep for children
who never know love or disaster.

VI

T-shirts tattooed with cartoon
animals, plastic smiles stretched
across your blossoming figure, remind
me you are becoming a woman.
Encase you in glass, protect
your bone china frame
from their hands. I raise you
in isolation, the chill too brutal
to remain outside. My heart dives
off cliffs chewing up the rabid tide.
God entrusted you to me
for protection. Guilt perforates my paper
heart like a sharpened pencil:
too lazy to read you a story
every night, got angry, pulled
just a bit tighter when I braided
your hair. I am sorry, my baby.
How could I let this happen?
I plead with Heaven, grant you
reprieve from the unforgiving.
If I don't find happiness, my girl,
what is a life?

Post Script: To those who stole my
daughter, run away, hide. I'm coming
to find her.

American Indian legends attribute the butterfly to a messenger between humanity and God. Legend states if one desires a wish to come true, capture a butterfly and whisper the wish to the winged creature. The butterfly, silent in its voice, cannot divulge the wish to anyone but the Great Spirit; therefore, when one releases the butterfly, it delivers the wish to heaven, a prayer carried on its wings. In gratitude for this kindness and for giving the creature freedom, the Great Spirit grants the wish—prayers answered.

Second Chances

A butterfly found me
in grass amongst clouds
of floating mushrooms and
dandelion orbs. I feared
its fate in my presence.
Every creature I touch
dies. I once suckled a Painted
Lady in petals pooled
with sweet nectar. I pulled its remains
from the mower weeks later,
caught between blade
and rotor, body crushed, wings
amber and black confetti
sprinkled in my hand. I crawled back
inside my pale cocoon, devastated
by the destruction. Now, I sit,
watch the butterfly stroke
its long black antennae and nuzzle
my hand. Fear does not occur
to it. Imagine what it feels like
to be a rose resurrected. Cherish
this moment—I'm alive. Such gifts
cannot be repeated.

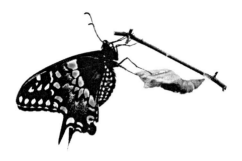

IV.

"You can stand me up at the gates of Hell, but I won't back down." —*Tom Petty and the Heartbreakers*

Who am I? My name is inconsequential, a tagline known only while I live. I am a daughter, sister unnoticed, wife, survivor, victim, child. I am a woman screaming, a writer, but above all else, I am a mother. Just like everyone else, I want to be remembered, not by my marbleized ideal, but by the imprint I leave upon the tapestry of humanity, the legacy born in my children. What mark do I leave in the wake of my daughter's ruination? How will her life impact the progression of society, the betterment of the world community, and the spiritual existence of others, as I so imagined long ago? Only time will tell the scope of her influence and the breadth of my voice as I send out evolutions of my authentic self through her laugh, her innocence, her corruption, her pain, and her smile.

Had I known my life would end up the way it has, and that motherhood would present me with such trying and difficult circumstances, I don't know if I would make the same decisions as I did. Yes, I question my choice to have children, not because I do not adore my daughters with every fiber of my being and would stop at nothing to provide them whatever they need, but I can't help but wonder what life had in store for me prior to Kamy's arrival. Like any other person who contemplates her existence, who wonders what missed opportunities lay scattered on the road not chosen, I ponder an independent life, a life not defined by my dependent child, but one fashioned of my own design. We do not get a choice; fate guides our feet as we traverse life. We have but two choices: fight our realities, forever struggling to survive a life not afforded to us, or accept destiny, submit to our calling, and live a prosperous, happy, and fulfilling existence given what God provides, for better or worse, for good or bad, in sickness and in health, to the most desperate and darkest of times, forever, Amen.

I don't have the answers. I search the world and heaven for reasons of my survival. Am I here to make others listen, to speak for those who fall silent, to stand for those who crumble? I seek the means to explain the enigma that is my life, and what I have learned is this: there are no secrets that require revealing, no master key that unlocks the centuries-old questions that plague humanity regarding the purpose of life, no cryptogram that deciphers the puzzle. The answer lies within, a simple and quiet solution burrowed deep inside the soul, a roar cloaked in a whisper, waiting for its unleashing into the still and stagnant air: the will and determination to persevere.

I dream of the exodus of the meek, the uprising of the forgotten. I want to arm legions with the most powerful weapon ever: their voice. I talk to Kamy about her illnesses; I educate and inform her so she remains enlightened to that which makes her special. I teach her to be an advocate for herself, to stand up for her rights and for the rights of all those who face the daunting task of living in our society with crippling mental illness; she has no choice. If she wants to lead any kind

of satisfying life, she must not only accept her fate, but celebrate it. She is broken, flawed, but she is mine, my darling little
girl who dreams of being an artist, who worships superheroes
and Peyton Manning, who fights the monsters set on consum-
ing her, who faces each day in the prison of her tortured mind
with bravery and wit, who wants so desperately just to be
included—my daughter. I don't know what the future holds
for Kamy, or me, or any of us. Life is uncertain, an undefined
amalgam ever shifting and changing. I do know, however,
that whatever obstacles we encounter, no matter how mighty
the storm, my daughter will not lose her grip. She came from
me—a survivor.

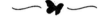

Moving Day

Life's skeletal remains
scatter about my floor,
signal endings in order
to begin again. I dig valuables
from closets and dresser drawers.
Cardboard boxes clog
my entryway, boxes left unpacked:
collected memories, pastoral
emulations, a frayed map of life's
last stages.

I can't go home.
It's grown too cold.
No one lives there
anymore. The roof caved
in long ago; I enter empty
rooms, find my other crouched
in a dark corner, weeping,
whittled down to bone. She follows
me into shadows; I only recognize her
going. The day becomes something
for which I have no name.
Hold onto memories
like a hole clings to light,
dream a house—
door open.

The Butterfly's Waltz

Dying caterpillar tucked inside
a suffocating shell.
Curled black tumor erupts,
paper body falls
away, aching from the metamorphosis.
Reborn a lovelier figure,
gold unfurls from flowering trees
a blizzard of wings
dropped from God's hand
onto my lips. Her name dances
away like a butterfly, ash
of my incinerated darling.
I have no choice;
life has a way of never stopping.

About the Author

Janna Vought is a published writer, with her works of poetry, short fiction, and nonfiction appearing in multiple literary journals and magazines. She is a graduate of Lindenwood University with an MFA in creative writing. She also is a 2013 AWP Intro Journals Nominee for poetry.

In addition to writing, Janna is also a doctoral candidate, working on her PhD in education. With this coursework, coupled with her nonprofit experience, she hopes to create a community outreach program that provides workshop experiences and creative writing courses for varying members of the community often ignored by mainstream academics, including the mentally ill and their families, victims of violent crime, at-risk youth, and other special populations who would benefit from learning about writing and implementing the craft in their own lives.

Her daughter, Kamryn, is diagnosed with bipolar I and Asperger's syndrome, an autism spectrum disorder, making her intimately qualified to write on parenting a special-needs child.

About Familius

Welcome to a place where mothers are celebrated, not compared. Where heart is at the center of our families, and family at the center of our homes. Where boo boos are still kissed, cake beaters are still licked, and mistakes are still okay. Welcome to a place where books—and family—are beautiful. Familius: a book publisher dedicated to helping families be happy.

Familius was founded in 2012 with the intent to align the founders' love of publishing and family with the digital publishing renaissance which occurred simultaneously with the Great Recession. The founders believe that the traditional family is the basic unit of society, and that a society is only as strong as the families that create it.

Familius's mission is to help families be happy. We invite you to participate with us in strengthening your family by being part of the Familius family. Go to www.familius.com to subscribe and receive information about our books, articles, and videos.

Website: www.familius.com
Facebook: www.facebook.com/paterfamilius
Twitter: @familiustalk, @paterfamilius1
Pinterest: www.pinterest.com/familius

CPSIA information can be obtained at www.ICGtesting.com
Printed in the USA
BVOW04s0409270913

332257BV00001B/1/P